EVIDENCE-BASED LEARNING STRATEGIES
FOR STUDENT PHARMACISTS

JAMES M. CULHANE
Professor and Assistant Dean for Student Academic Success Programs
Notre Dame of Maryland University School of Pharmacy
Baltimore, Maryland

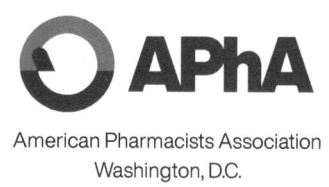

American Pharmacists Association
Washington, D.C.

Notice:

The authors and publisher have made every effort to ensure the accuracy and completeness of the information presented in this book. However, the authors and publisher cannot be held responsible for the continued currency of the information, any inadvertent errors or omissions, or the application of this information. Therefore, the authors and publisher shall have no liability to any person or entity with regard to claims, loss, or damage caused or alleged to be caused, directly or indirectly, by the use of information contained herein.

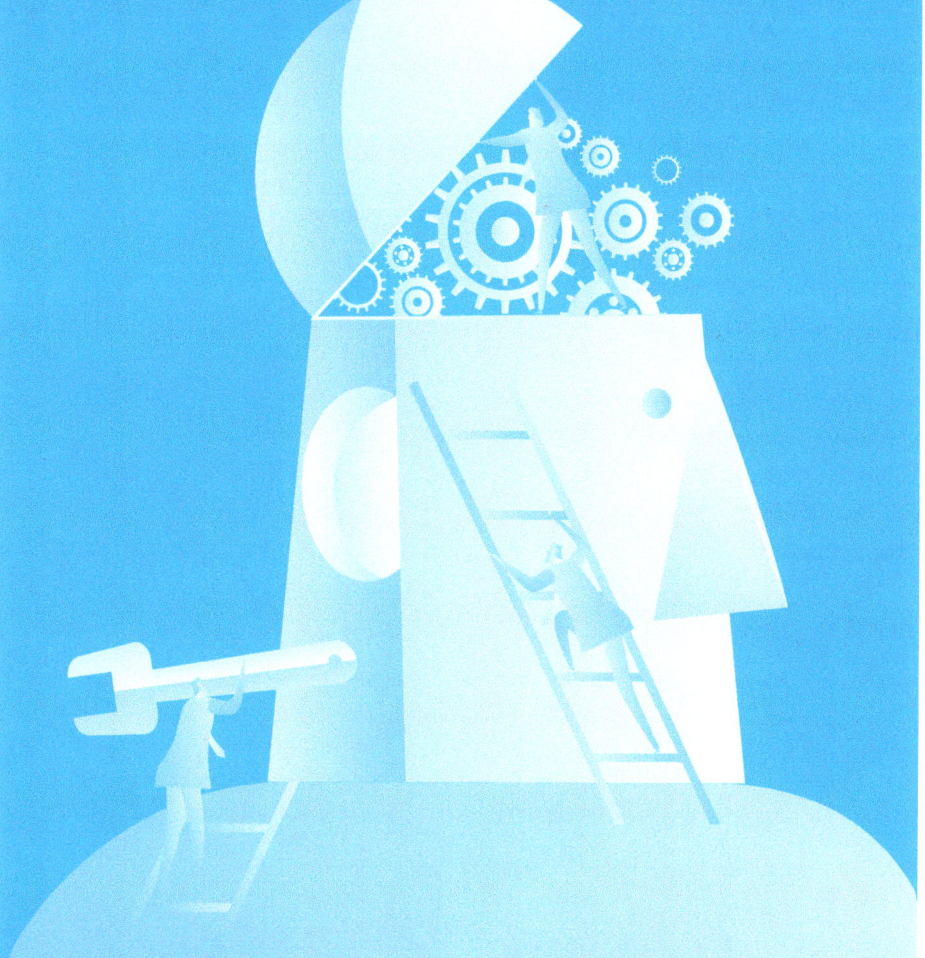

EVIDENCE-BASED LEARNING STRATEGIES FOR STUDENT PHARMACISTS

JAMES M. CULHANE

APhA

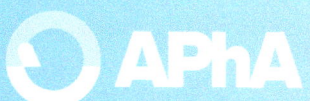

Senior Director, Books and Digital Publishing: Eleanore Tapscott
Editorial Director: Jesse Vineyard
Production Editor: Brittany Williams
Editorial Services: Circle Graphics, Inc.
Cover Design: Jane DeBruijn, APhA Integrated Design and Production

©2022 by the American Pharmacists Association
APhA was founded in 1852 as the American Pharmaceutical Association.

Published by the American Pharmacists Association
2215 Constitution Avenue, NW
Washington, DC 20037-2985
www.pharmacist.com
www.pharmacylibrary.com

All rights reserved

No part of this publication may be reproduced, stored in a retrieval system, or transmitted in any form or by any means, electronic, mechanical, photocopying, recording, or otherwise, without written permission from the publisher.

To comment on this book by e-mail, send your message to the publisher at aphabooks@aphanet.org.

Library of Congress Cataloging-in-Publication Data available upon request.

How to Order This Book
Online: www.pharmacist.com/shop
By phone: 800-878-0729 (770-280-0085 from outside the United States)
VISA®, MasterCard®, and American Express® cards accepted.

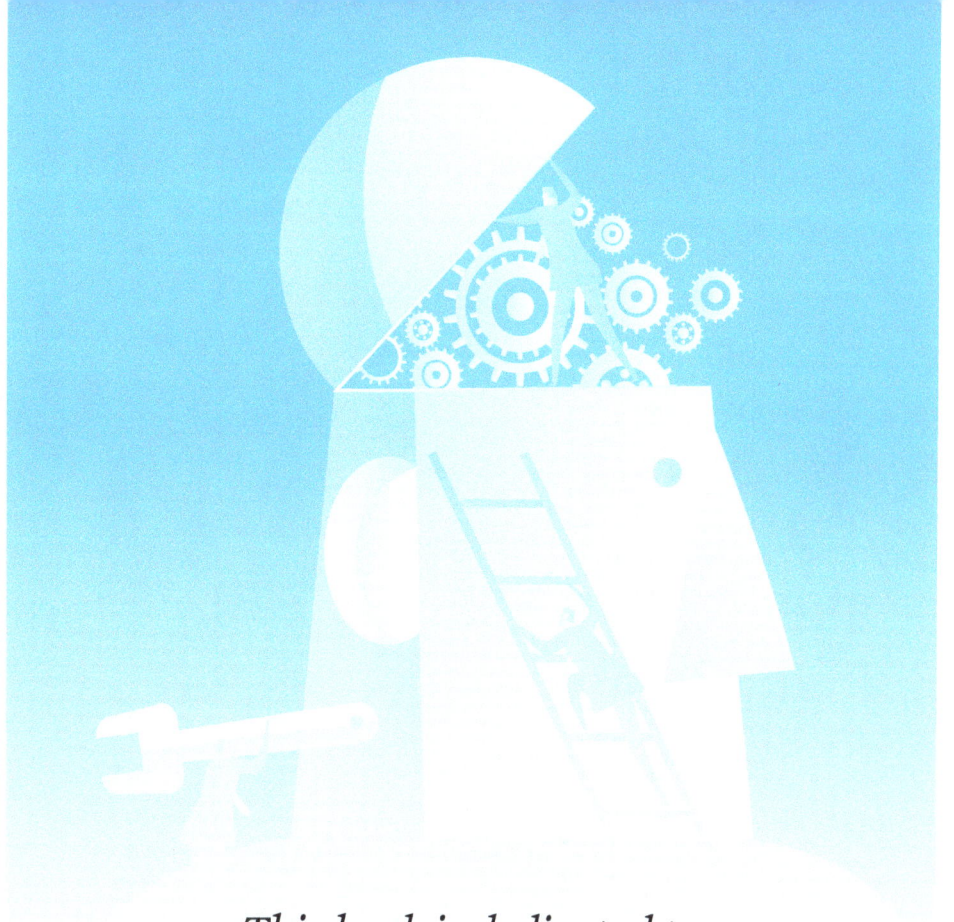

This book is dedicated to any pharmacy student who has ever struggled academically, felt like they were just trying to survive or questioned their ability to graduate from pharmacy school.

Hang in there. You've got this!

CONTENTS

INTRODUCTION .... **IX**

CHAPTER 1 - Metacognition, Evidenced-Based Learning Strategies, and the S.A.L.A.M.I. Method **01**

CHAPTER 2 - Learning Goals **13**

CHAPTER 3 - Productivity **21**

CHAPTER 4 - S.A.L.A.M.I. Method Step 1: Preclass Preparation **41**

CHAPTER 5 - S.A.L.A.M.I. Method Step 2: In-Class Engagement **55**

CHAPTER 6 - S.A.L.A.M.I. Method Step 3: Postclass Review **71**

CHAPTER 7 - S.A.L.A.M.I. Method Step 4: Preexam Preparation Part 1, Keys to Effective Studying **79**

CHAPTER 8 - S.A.L.A.M.I. Method Step 4: Preexam Preparation Part 2, Active Recall Strategies **95**

CHAPTER 9 - S.A.L.A.M.I. Method Step 5: Postassessment Review .. **127**

CHAPTER 10 - Final Thoughts **143**

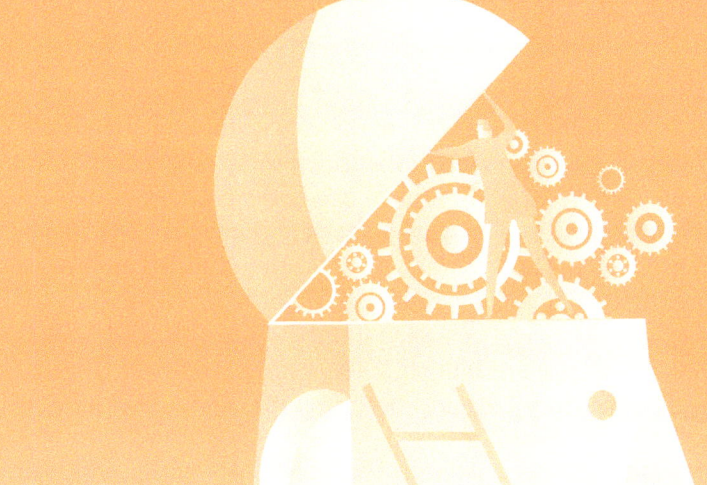

INTRODUCTION

"Intention to learn is helpful only if it leads to the use of good learning strategies."

— **Alan Baddeley**

I'd like to ask you some questions.

> 1. Have you ever failed an exam or performed poorly in a course and knew you could do better?
>
> 2. Have you ever felt completely overwhelmed and anxious about your academic course load?
>
> 3. Are you unsure that you will be able to learn all you need to care successfully for patients?

If you answered yes to any of these questions, then I know exactly how you feel. I'd also like to offer some help.

Let's face it, being a pharmacy student is tough. In my 25 years as a pharmacy professor, I have witnessed significant changes in the educational demands placed on students. Driven by the rapid advances in the biological, pharmaceutical, and clinical sciences as well as the expanding clinical role of the pharmacist in all practice settings, pharmacy schools have had to make substantial changes to their curricula. These include expanding already crowded didactic and experiential elements and adding extensive cocurricular and extracurricular requirements for graduation. To graduate, pharmacy students must be able to navigate all of this while still meeting personal and work-related responsibilities. It sounds impossible, and for many students it presents a significant challenge, especially if they have difficulty learning.

There are many reasons why students struggle with their learning. Some are unsuccessful because they lack necessary prerequisite knowledge or experience. Others may not reach their potential due to socioeconomic challenges or health-related issues. Still others fall short due to lack of appropriate motivation or solid learning skills. I am familiar with what it is like to be a struggling student because I was one. In high school, I earned good grades, participated in all the "right" extracurricular activities, and chose a local college with an excellent reputation. I majored in chemistry in hopes of fulfilling my dreams of attending medical school. Unfortunately, my first 2 years in college were less than successful. By the time I entered my junior year, it began to dawn on me (thanks to my middling academic performance and the recent letter I received from the college's prehealth committee) that my life's career plan was about to change, whether I wanted it to or not. I was devastated, lost, and confused. Fortunately, I had some good academic advising and a wonderful winter internship that led me to a graduate program in Pharmacology and Toxicology.

Considering what I just revealed about myself, I am certain that the irony of finding myself on the first day of graduate school sitting in a physiology course with 80+ first-year medical students will not be lost on you. The scene that day was what you might expect. Some students were sitting, some were standing, and others were milling about waiting for their first lecture to begin. It was abundantly clear from facial expressions and tone of background conversations that the emotions in the room were a mix of anticipation, excitement, and a heavy dose of anxiety. Speaking for myself, I was panicked and felt a little like a fraud. The hard lesson I had learned from my undergraduate experience was that I was not smart enough to go to medical school and that I had no idea how I was going to pass this course.

Promptly at 8:00 AM our professor walked into the front of the classroom. As students quickly found their seats, he silently set down his lecture notes, dimmed the lights, and turned on the overhead projector. Turning towards the class, he stood for a moment looking out across the lecture hall. Silence fell across the across the room, and as we sat, pens ready and notebooks open, he spoke the words that would have a profound impact on my life.

> *"Studying for medical school is like eating a salami."*

What I most remember from that moment was confusion. As I looked at my fellow classmates out of the corner of my eye to gauge their reactions, I remember thinking, "What did salami have to do with physiology or studying for medical school?" The only thing I really knew about salami was that it was a deli meat and delicious when eaten on a bagel with cream cheese. I could tell from my classmate's facial expressions and murmuring that I was not alone in my confusion. As the whispered confusion subsided, our professor went on to explain his statement to the class. His explanation is best summarized from the following excerpt taken from a worksheet passed out in class that morning:

> *"You study material daily in small, manageable portions just as you would eat —and digest!— 'salami slices' in daily meals as opposed to swallowing the whole salami in a single meal on the weekend."*

This worksheet also contained a "recipe for an efficient learning strategy" and was based on an article recently published in the journal Academic Medicine.[1] This "recipe" required the use of the following 6 "ingredients":

1. **previewing material and notes the night before lecture**
2. **taking notes in class**
3. **studying and correcting class notes on the same day**
4. **getting daily feedback through self-testing**
5. **getting timely help from instructors**
6. **reinforcing and cleaning up problem areas on the weekend**

That evening I began to consider what I learned in class, and it began to dawn on me that perhaps the reason for my underperformance as an undergraduate was my approach to learning was faulty. I had survived largely through sheer will and determination, suffering through long, last-minute cramming sessions and using passive study strategies that looked nothing like the proposed method I had learned that day. As I committed to apply the basic principles of this "methodology," I began to see immediate improvement in my learning. Daily structured studying of material in small manageable bites, while still challenging, began reaping rewards far more important than just good grades. For the first time, I felt free to learn material for the sake of learning, not just to pass a course. Any anxiety that I had in the past about academic success was overshadowed by my new ability to retain and apply concepts that I was learning.

Despite the profound impact this strategy had on my learning, I do not want to give the false impression that it made school easy or that I did not experience challenges and struggles. Real learning is hard work. Like any student, I suffered normal pretest anxiety, studied long hours, and sometimes wondered if classes would ever end. I even had a few bad exams. The difference was that I had a system and a set of skills that gave me the confidence to tackle any academic challenge no matter how difficult.

The members of the medical physiology teaching team and my professors in the Pharmacology and Toxicology Department where I earned my PhD were exceptional educators. They realized that good teaching was more than just effective transferal of information to their students. They saw it as an opportunity to teach students how to learn. Moreover, they were able to translate and operationalize the latest (at the time) learning theory so that it was useful to their students. I hope that with this book I can carry on this legacy.

Much has been learned about human learning since I was a graduate student. Recent advances in the field of cognitive psychology have revealed powerful, evidence-based learning strategies that teachers and students can use to increase retention and understanding of new information. Books like *Make it Stick: The Science of Successful Learning; A Mind for Numbers: How to Excel at Science and Math; Learn Better: Mastering the Skills for Success in Life, Business, and School, or How to Become an Expert in Just About Anything;*[2-3] and web-based resources like The Learning Scientists' website and podcast (https://www.learningscientists.org/podcast-episodes)[4] and the extremely popular Massive Online Open Course (MOOC) "Learning How to Learn"[5] are just a few of the many examples of how scientists and educators are trying to spread the word about evidence-based learning strategies and to debunk some of the myths we hold about learning. The dissemination of these findings are coming in the nick of time as students are experiencing a crisis in higher education. Tuition costs continue to rise while completion rates of 4-year degrees in the United States are abysmally low with only 54% of undergraduate students completing a 4-year degree in 6 years.[6] Data collected by the American Association of Colleges of Pharmacy (AACP) in their annual Profile of Pharmacy Students reveals that pharmacy student attrition rates have steadily risen from a low of 1.3% in 2004 to over 12% in 2019, with 6.7% of pharmacy students experiencing delayed graduation.[7]

The systematized approach to learning described in this book is largely based on these learning strategies, as well as fundamental and proven teaching principles, the best advice from learning experts, and my own personal experience as a teacher and academic coach. It is designed to be a practical guide to help students that lack an organized approach to their studying and to help those that do, improve their effectiveness as learners. Over my career, I have seen firsthand the psychological and financial consequences of delayed graduation, dismissal, or withdrawals on student pharmacists. While some of these students had confounding factors that could not be helped, I believe that many might have had a different outcome if they had possessed the necessary skills and knowledge about effective learning strategies. I hope that the strategies in this book in partnership with your effort and commitment will help you avoid becoming a statistic and develop into an effective and independent life-long learner.

REFERENCES

1. Norman GR, Schmidt HG. The psychological basis of problem-based learning. *Acad Med.* 1992;67(9):557-565.
2. Brown PC, Roediger III, HL, McDaniel, MA. *Make It Stick: The Science of Successful Learning.* Cambridge, MA: The Belknap Press of Harvard University Press; 2014.
3. Oakley B. A Mind for Numbers: *How to Excel at Math and Science (Even If You Flunked Algebra).* New York, NY: Jeremy P. Tarcher/Penguin; 2014.
4. The Learning Scientists. Available at: https://www.learningscientists.org. Accessed February 24, 2022.
5. Massive Online Open Course (MOOC). Learning how to learn: Powerful mental tools to help you master tough subjects. Available at: https://www.my-mooc.com/en/mooc/learning-how-to-learn/. Accessed February 24, 2022.
6. Shapiro D, Dundar A, Huie F, Wakhungu P, Bhimdiwala A, Wilson SE. *Completing College: Eight Year Completion Outcomes for the Fall 2010 Cohort. Supplemental Feature. (Signature Report No. 12c).* Herndon, VA: National Student Clearinghouse Research Center; 2019.
7. American Associations of Colleges of Pharmacy. 2018-2019 Annual Survey of Pharmacy Students. Available at: https://www.aacp.org/sites/default/files/2020-05/fall-2019-pps-degrees-conferred.pdf. Accessed January 25, 2022.

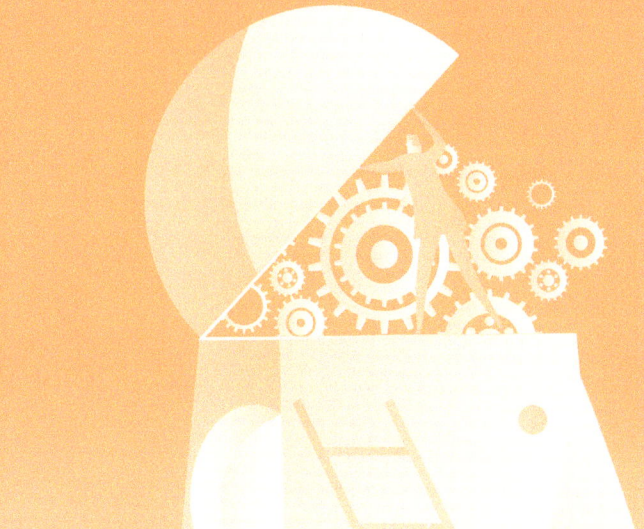

CHAPTER 1
Metacognition, Evidenced-Based Learning Strategies, and the S.A.L.A.M.I. Method

Before we dive into some of the concepts in this chapter, let's take a few minutes to examine the following case study. As you read through the case study ask yourself the following questions:

1. To which aspects of C.M.'s situation do you relate?

2. Can you identify any clues that might be the cause of C.M.'s poor academic performance?

Case Study

C.M. is a second-year pharmacy student who comes to me with concerns about poor course performance. As an undergraduate, C.M. earned A's and B's in science courses and found them to be "relatively simple." Since entering pharmacy school, C.M. has struggled to get C's in most courses and is in danger of failing one this semester. C.M. describes working "really hard", studying four to six hours per day and all day on Saturday and Sunday. The majority of C.M.'s study time is spent reading and highlighting course textbooks and recopying notes. C.M. is frustrated and can't understand why this approach to studying, which worked in high school and undergraduate courses, is no longer effective.

CASE STUDY ANALYSIS

It may surprise you that many students like C.M., who were strong performers in undergraduate science courses, can struggle in a highly demanding professional degree program. Even though C.M. is a smart, well-intentioned, and motivated learner who devotes a significant amount of time to studying, the likely hood of this student improving in academic performance is low. Without some type of intervention, one of two outcomes are likely to occur. C.M. will either continue to fail courses and end up on academic probation or, in a worst-case scenario, get dismissed from the program. The alternative outcome is that C.M. will end up, through trial and error, figuring out a learning strategy that will help achieve the minimum grades that will allow progression through the program. Neither outcome is desirable. Examination of some of the clues in this scenario might help to make sense of what is going on with C.M. and may provide some insight into your own learning challenges.

The first clue that stands out to me is the disconnect between the amount of time C.M. is spending on studying and the grades earned. Based on our conversation it appears that C.M. is spending about 45 hours per week studying. This should be more than enough time to achieve good grades, provided that (1) the student's estimation of study time is accurate, (2) there are no apparent learning disabilities, and (3) the techniques and approaches being used to study are evidence-based. The second and third clues are closely related and are reflected by the student's prerequisite science course grades and methodologies used for studying. As an undergraduate, C.M. appeared to be a capable science student. Based on this prior success, C.M. decides to use the same study techniques in pharmacy school that worked before. This is an approach that I see often in the students that I coach, and more often than not it leads to poor grades.

C.M. continues to use the minimally effective study strategies like rereading and highlighting the text and recopying notes. While these strategies were effective enough to allow for good performance in C.M.'s undergraduate science courses, they are overwhelmed by the level of difficulty and sheer amount of material that needs to be mastered in a highly demanding professional degree program. As the poor grades begin to accumulate and the frustration and despair mounts, students like C.M. tend to "dig in" and try to improve their performance by doing more of the same. Unfortunately, this rarely works. For C.M. to be successful, acquisition of new learning skills and approaches will be needed.

Metacognition

Take a few minutes and study the list below. How many of the strategies listed have you used in your course work?

- **Rereading the text, class notes, handouts, or PowerPoint® slides.**
- **Studying highlighted material in the text.**
- **Waiting to study for an exam several days before the test.**
- **Waiting until several days before an exam to do practice or application problems.**
- **Participating in a study group that does more socializing than studying.**
- **Rewatching or relistening to recorded lectures.**
- **Recopying notes.**
- **Condensing and then memorizing your notes.**
- **Studying one topic for several hours and not revisiting that material for several days.**

If you are reading this book, my guess is that you have used at least one of these approaches, and you are not alone. Numerous studies have demonstrated that students in very diverse academic settings and programs, including pharmacy, tend to prefer these low-impact strategies.[1-6]

Now let's consider an even more important set of questions.

1. **Do I often think that I know more than my grades reflect?**
2. **Does the use of my study strategies allow me to accomplish specific goals during my study session or do I use them based on habit, convenience, or a lack of knowing what else to do?**
3. **Does the use of my study strategies benefit my understanding, long-term retention, and ability to apply information?**
4. **Do I regularly use active or passive study strategies?**

Your answers to these questions are extremely important as they are the key to understanding why you study the way that you do and the probability that you will achieve your academic goals.

Loosely defined, metacognition is an awareness or understanding of how one thinks and learns.[7] While metacognition might sound like an amazing ability possessed by a superhero, it is a skill that can be developed, leading to significant improvement in your learning. In fact, numerous scientific articles suggest that students with a high degree of metacognitive awareness and skills tend to be more independent and successful in their learning.[8-10]

There are three aspects of metacognition that every pharmacy student can develop and use to help improve learning. These include developing a basic understanding of metacognition, learning how to monitor the progress of learning, and picking and choosing appropriate strategies to maximize learning.[11] Applying these aspects to your own learning is critical in becoming an independent learner who can quickly and effectively acquire knowledge, retain that knowledge, and retrieve that knowledge from memory to solve problems, pass exams, and effectively care for patients. It is also a primary goal of this book.

Metacognitive knowledge encompasses what we know and believe about our own learning. Learning about effective, evidence-based learning strategies and dispelling the many myths about effective studying is one way to develop in this area. As mentioned previously, there are numerous studies demonstrating that students tend to prefer using inefficient learning strategies while studying. These studies correlate well to my own experience as an academic coach. I have found that students frequently choose to use these strategies because they don't know any better. When I introduce them to evidence-based approaches like active recall and teach them how to incorporate them in their study, significant improvements in their learning follows.

Metacognitive monitoring involves regularly assessing the effectiveness of your learning. Leading experts in the field of cognitive psychology have discovered that "our intuitions and introspections appear to be unreliable as a guide to how we should manage our own learning activities."[12] In other words, human beings are very poor at gauging how well or how much we have learned. If you have ever been disappointed with a grade on an exam that you felt well prepared for, you know what I mean. Monitoring the effectiveness of your daily learning by generating and analyzing actual data while you study, rather than relying on your "feelings of learning" can help you to be more efficient by avoiding over- and underlearning. If you are overconfident in your learning of a particular concept, you might not study it enough. If you are underconfident, you might spend more time learning it than necessary.[13] Additionally, the data can also be an important indicator of when you need to change your approach to studying. In Chapter 8, I will explain a study strategy called "the boxing technique" that will help you to do this.

Metacognitive control requires that you can regulate specific components of your learning by adopting and adapting evidence-based practices. If adapting a brand-new study strategy seems frightening or intimidating, you are not alone. Many of the students I have worked with have struggled to let go of their own preconceived ideas about what study skills and strategies work. Changing your approach to learning requires a conscious effort to go against feelings and intuition, confront fear of failure, and examine preconceived ideas about learning. Once you do, the benefits are significant. A recent article published in the *American Journal of Pharmaceutical Education* highlights this point by encouraging faculty to work with students to develop metacognitive knowledge, awareness, and control and by arguing that students who have a high degree of metacognitive awareness perform better academically.[14]

So how do you know if you possess a high level of metacognitive awareness? There are a number of questionnaires that are available to help you to gauge this; however, I think these are best used in conjunction with a faculty member or learning specialist that will help you to assess the results and formulate a plan for improvement.[14] Based on these questionnaires I have generated the following list of student behaviors and characteristics. Read through them and consider whether you engage in any of these behaviors. When you are studying outside of class, do you

1. **Consistently evaluate the effectiveness of your study environments and actively monitor and avoid procrastination?**
2. **Set goals for studying?**
3. **Implement evidence-based study strategies like active recall, spacing, and elaboration?**
4. **Monitor your daily learning through self-testing?**
5. **Use the results of daily self-testing and performance on classroom activities, quizzes, and exams to determine accurately the extent of your learning and adjust how and what you are studying?**

If you use one or more of these approaches, you possess some of the knowledge and skills necessary for effective learning. If not, keep reading! As you move through your academic training, continuing to develop metacognitive behaviors and skills that match the learning challenges you will face is important. In subsequent chapters we will take a deeper look at strategies and tools specifically designed to encourage the development of these skills and to help you use the five strategies listed above in your daily learning.

Evidence-Based Learning Strategies

In the previously cited studies, most students choose to use low-impact, inefficient learning strategies like rereading, highlighting, condensing, and recopying notes when they are studying. The reasons for this are complex but generally involve a lack of knowledge of effective learning strategies and of how to implement them in their daily study. Replacing these strategies with evidence-based ones is a key to your academic success. There are at least seven to eight evidence-based learning strategies that show significant promise and are applicable to the type of learning you do as a pharmacy student.[15] Of these, I have picked the most effective and relevant strategies: active recall, spacing, interleaving, and elaboration.

ACTIVE RECALL

Active recall, also known as self-testing, retrieval practice, and practice testing, is one of the top evidence-based learning strategies that you can use.[16] There is a significant body of scientific literature that supports its effectiveness, and I have seen amazing changes in learning and grades in students who effectively apply this strategy.[17] Learning to use active recall in your study is as simple as trying to remember facts and information that you have previously studied. There are many ways to use active recall in your study, and I will explain several of my favorites in Chapter 8. In fact, I think active recall is so important that if you took away only one lesson from this entire book, it should be how to use active recall in your study.

SPACING

Spacing is another extremely powerful, yet simple, evidence-based learning strategy, and its benefits have been well documented in the scientific literature.[18,19] Unfortunately, most students I work with do not use this approach initially. They are already engaged in either massed or blocked studying. Massed studying, often referred to as cramming, is the most common approach I see with my students. It involves studying intensely right before an exam. Blocking study is another common strategy in which students choose to spend the weekly time allotted to study a topic in one or two study sessions during the week. These two approaches are not optimal for learning and long-term retention of material. Spacing involves studying for a class at regular intervals throughout the week. An example of using spacing in your study would be to study a subject for one hour every day of the week. Spacing is most effective when it is coupled to retrieval practice or active recall. When the two of these approaches are used simultaneously it is referred to as distributed practice. You will learn more about the spacing effect and how to apply it to your daily study in Chapter 7.

INTERLEAVING

Interleaving is one of the more challenging evidence-based learning strategies to describe. Simply put it is mixing or interweaving similar concepts together as you study.[20]

Interleaving can be used with many aspects of your learning strategies to include planning your study sessions and engaging in active recall and problem solving.

Interleaving can be a great strategy to use when planning a study session. Instead of studying only one subject during a three-hour study session (blocking), mix it up and study several subjects for shorter periods of time. Every time you switch to a new subject your brain has to mentally shift gears, reintroducing a desirable difficulty.

When engaging in active recall during study, there are several ways to incorporate interleaving. The first involves mixing up material that you are self-testing. A great example of when interleaving can be used effectively involves a recall task with which most pharmacy students are familiar, learning the top 200 prescribed drugs. In my experience, students commonly use flashcards for self-testing while studying the drugs. When self-testing, the flashcards can be grouped by therapeutic and/or pharmacological class. For example, if you are studying the top prescribed antihypertensive medications, you might first work through all of the angiotensin-converting-enzyme (ACE) inhibitor cards and then move on to the calcium channel blockers, followed by beta antagonists. After several times through the deck, you will probably find that you are quickly becoming familiar with each one of the drugs. Now, let's shuffle all the antihypertensive drug cards, so that they are no longer grouped based on their mechanism of action and began testing yourself again. I suspect that you would find remembering much more difficult. This is interleaving. The benefit of interleaving is that it introduces a positive level of difficulty to your studying, which appears to strengthen learning. This is known as a "desirable difficulty."[21] If you want to further increase the level of difficulty, mix the antihypertensive drugs in with those used to treat diabetes.

Another example involves mixing active recall of subjects that you are studying during the same study session. For example, let's say that you are planning on spending 30 minutes practicing active recall on your pharmacology course and the next 30 minutes on your therapeutics course. Mix the two together and switch back and forth between them during the same study session.

If you are working on solving problems in pharmaceutics or pharmacokinetics, don't attempt to solve a group of similar problems in one setting. Mix the problems up so that you must switch between different problem types. This will help you to learn how to choose and apply the right method for each of the problem types rather than just learning the method itself.[22] As you can see, they are many creative ways of using interleaving when you study, and it can be a very effective strategy to enhance your learning, especially when combined with active recall and elaboration.

ELABORATION

Of all the evidence-based learning strategies, elaboration is probably the one with which you are most familiar. Many of my students report using this strategy in their daily studying without realizing it is an evidence-based approach. If you have sat in an empty room and explained concepts to yourself, you have used elaboration. If you have every studied in a group and explained concepts to your classmates, you have used elaboration. If you have ever tried to explain pharmacogenomics to your cat, you have used elaboration. In the context of studying, elaboration is simply explaining concepts that you are trying to learn in your own words and with as many details as possible.[23] A form of elaboration about which we will talk extensively in Chapter 7 is elaborative interrogation. This form of elaboration goes a little deeper and involves asking who, what, why, where, when, or how questions about the material you are studying. It also involves making connections, comparing and contrasting the concept you are learning with other related concepts.[24]

S.A.L.A.M.I.: Systematic Approach to Learning and Metacognitive Improvement

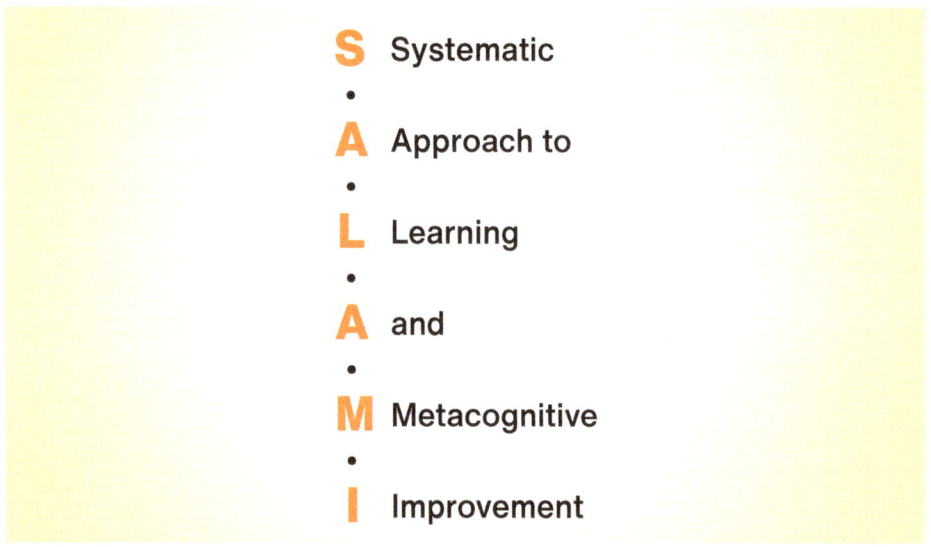

Figure 1-1: S.A.L.A.M.I. Acronym

The acronym S.A.L.A.M.I. stands for a systematic approach to learning and metacognitive improvement. The S.A.L.A.M.I. method is designed to help students improve their learning through the use of evidence-based learning strategies and best practices and to increase their ability to successfully self-regulate their learning (metacognition).

This acronym is a tribute to the analogy I learned as a graduate student and highlights two major focal points of the method. The first is to help you become an independent and self-directed learner with a high degree of metacognitive knowledge, monitoring, and control. The second is to teach you how to use practically the evidence-based learning strategies I have mentioned above. Achieving these goals will require you to become familiar with the process of learning; to master the use of evidenced-based, high-impact learning strategies; and to work to develop metacognitive awareness, specifically the ability to self-assess, monitor, and regulate how you learn.[25]

As I was researching the method, I was inspired by Anders Ericsson's and Robert Pool's book, *Peak: Secrets from the New Science of Expertise*. Accomplished people in every field and endeavor have used the techniques and processes they describe to develop expertise. In this book, Ericsson and Pool make a compelling argument that the key feature of being successful in any task or discipline is not natural ability but rather the practice process used by the individual to develop expertise.[26] They also argue that if the right approach is taken, developing expertise in a field is attainable by almost anyone. I wholeheartedly agree with this, especially when it comes to students and learning. I have seen student's transform their academic performance when they begin to adopt an approach similar to what Ericsson and Pool recommend.

Ericsson and Pool describe three different types of practice that can be used when learning new information or skills. These are naïve, purposeful, and deliberate practice. Naïve practice is based on the belief that doing something over and over can help you master a skill or body of knowledge. This approach may sound familiar to you as this is the most common study approach used by my students. I know that an intervention is necessary when I hear my students emphatically promise that they will study harder and longer for the next exam after just having received a poor grade, especially when using low-impact study strategies like rereading or re-copying notes. The next type, purposeful practice, requires repetition and feedback from performances to determine if there are deficiencies in skills or knowledge so that they can be corrected. When applied to studying, this type of practice requires that you have an overarching plan to prepare for the upcoming assessment, create and follow daily well-defined and specific study goals, devote your full attention to study-related activities, use evidence-based learning strategies in your study, and consistently assess and make changes to your practice based on your assessment performance. This type of practice requires metacognitive awareness, and while it is far superior to naïve practice, it does have its limitations, especially when a plateau in performance is reached.

Deliberate practice is designed to help you break through this plateau, and, while it shares many of the characteristics of purposeful practice, it differs in that it requires the intervention of a teacher or expert to guide your practice. Ideally, professors and instructors can serve in this capacity provided they are experts in the content area that you are learning and possess a working knowledge of effective techniques that enhance acquisition, retention, and application of knowledge. While this is an ideal situation it does not often play out in real life because of two major reasons. The first is that while professors are content experts in the fields in which they teach, many are unfamiliar with how to coach students in the process of learning. Secondly, students are often hesitant to seek help from their professors, fearing that they will look incompetent or lazy. If you feel that you require expertise in learning how to learn, many colleges and universities have learning centers that can assist you. In addition, there are academic coaches like me, who are available to work with you on an individual basis if needed. If none of these options are available to you, I hope that this book can provide you with some direction.

The S.A.L.A.M.I. method is designed around the typical, daily learning experiences (before, during, and after class) to mirror your didactic courses. Specific learning and metacognitive techniques are employed during each of the steps to help students use their time efficiently and to maximize learning. Over subsequent pages we will explore in detail the various steps of the S.A.L.A.M.I. method, which include

1. **Preclass preparation**
2. **In-class engagement**
3. **Postclass evaluation**
4. **Encoding and consolidation**
5. **Postassessment review**

While the techniques and skills presented in each step of the S.A.L.A.M.I. method can be used on their own, they are most effective when used in conjunction with one another. At first many of the strategies in the S.A.L.A.M.I. method may seem awkward, counterintuitive, or even unproductive. That's normal. Breaking old habits can be difficult, and developing new skills can take time. Like any endeavor focused on self-improvement, do not expect immediate results. Behavior changes and skill development takes time, but the long-term payoff is significant!

Key Concepts from Chapter 1

1. **Academic success requires students to**
   a. **work on the development of metacognitive knowledge, monitoring, and control.**
   b. **consistently use evidence-based learning strategies in their daily studies.**
   c. **use performance data generated by active recall, learning activities, and assessments—not feelings—to gauge the effectiveness of their learning.**

2. There are many evidence-based learning strategies that can be used to enhance learning. These include active recall, spacing, interleaving, and elaboration.

3. Many students use ineffective study strategies. They do this because of a false belief that these strategies work or because they just don't know any better.

4. Real learning is hard work. No study strategy will change that; however, using effective study strategies can help you get more out of your study sessions and improve your learning and academic performance.

REFERENCES

1. Kornell N, Bjork RA. The promise and perils of self-regulated study. *Psychon Bull Rev.* 2007;14(2):219-224. doi:10.3758/BF03194055.
2. Yan VX, Thai KP, Bjork RA. Habits and beliefs that guide self-regulated learning: do they vary with mindset? *J Appl Res Mem Cogn.* 2014;3(3):140-152. doi:10.1016/j.jarmac.2014.04.003.
3. Hartwig MK, Dunlosky J. Study strategies of college students: Are self-testing and scheduling related to achievement? *Psychon Bull Rev.* 2012;19(1):126-134. doi:10.3758/s13423-011-0181-y.
4. Geller J, Toftness AR, Armstrong PI, et al. Study strategies and beliefs about learning as a function of academic achievement and achievement goals. *Memory.* 2018;26(5):683-690. doi:10.1080/09658211.2017.1397175.
5. McAndrew M. Dental student study strategies: are self-testing and scheduling related to academic performance? *J Dent Education.* 2016;8(5):542-552.
6. Persky AM, Hudson SL. A snapshot of student study strategies across a professional pharmacy curriculum: are students using evidence-based practice? *Curr Pharm Teach Learn.* 2016;8(2):141-147. doi:10.1016/j.cptl.2015.12.010.
7. Flavell JH. Metacognition and cognitive monitoring a new area of cognitive-developmental Inquiry. *Am Psychol.* 1979;34(10):906-991.
8. Hartman HJ. *Metacognition in Learning and Instruction: Theory, Research and Practice.* Dordrecht, The Netherlands: Kluwer Academic Publishers; 2001.
9. Bailey H, Dunlosky J, Hertzog C. Metacognitive training at home: does it improve older adults' learning? *Gerontology.* 2010;56(4):414-420. doi:10.1159/000266030.
10. Stewart D, Panus P, Hagemeier N, Thigpen J, Brooks L. Pharmacy student self-testing as a predictor of examination performance. *Am J Pharm Edu.* 2014;78(2)32.doi.org/10.5688/ajpe78232.
11. Dunlosky J, Metcalfe J. *Metacognition.* Los Angeles, CA: SAGE Publications, Inc.; 2008.
12. Bjork RA, Dunlosky J, Kornell N. Self-regulated learning: beliefs, techniques, and illusions. *Annu Rev Psychol.* 2013;64(1):417-444.
13. Dunlosky J, Rawson KA. Overconfidence produces underachievement: inaccurate self-evaluations undermine students' learning and retention. *Learn Instr.* 2012;22(4):271-280. doi:10.1016/j.learninstruc.2011.08.003.
14. Rivers ML, Dunlosky J, Persky AM. Measuring metacognitive knowledge, monitoring, and control in the pharmacy classroom and experiential settings. *Am J Pharm Educ.* 2020;84(5):7730. doi:10.5688/ajpe7730.

15. Dunlosky J, Rawson KA, Marsh EJ, Nathan MJ, Willingham DT. Improving students' learning with effective learning techniques: promising directions from cognitive and educational psychology. *Psychol Sci Public Interest*. 2013;14(1):4-58. doi:10.1177/1529100612453266.
16. Abbott EE. On the analysis of the factors of recall in the learning process. *The Psychological Review: Monograph Supplements*. 1909;11(1):159-177.
17. Karpicke JD, Roediger HL. The critical importance of retrieval for learning. *Science*. 2008;319(5865):966-968. doi:10.1126/science.1152408.
18. Cepeda NJ, Pashler H, Vul E, Wixted JT, Rohrer D. Distributed practice in verbal recall tasks: a review and quantitative synthesis. *Psychol Bull*. 2006;132(3):354-380. doi:10.1037/0033-2909.132.3.354.
19. Carpenter SK, Cepeda NJ, Rohrer D, Kang SHK, Pashler H. Using spacing to enhance diverse forms of learning: review of recent research and implications for instruction. *Educ Psychol Rev*. 2012;24(3):369-378. doi:10.1007/s10648-012-9205-z.
20. Rohrer D. Interleaving helps students distinguish among similar concepts. *Educ Psychol Rev*. 2012;24(3):355-367. doi:10.1007/s10648-012-9201-3.
21. Metcalfe J, Shimamura AP, eds. Memory and Metamemory Considerations in the Training of Human Beings. In: *Metacognition*. The MIT Press; 1994:185-205. doi:10.7551/mitpress/4561.003.0011.
22. Weinstein Y, Madan CR, Sumeracki MA. Teaching the science of learning. *Cogn Res Princ Implic*. 2018;3(1):2. doi:10.1186/s41235-017-0087-y.
23. Chi MTH, De Leeuw N, Chiu MH, Lavancher C. Eliciting self-explanations improves understanding. *Cogn Sci*. 1994;18(3):439-477. doi:10.1207/s15516709cog1803_3.
24. McDaniel M, Donnelly CM. Learning with analogy and elaborative interrogation. *J Educ Psychol*. 1996;88:508-519. doi:10.1037/0022-0663.88.3.508.
25. Schunk DH. Self-efficacy and academic motivation. *Educ Psychol*. 1991;26:207-223.
26. Ericsson A, Pool R. *Peak: Secrets from the New Science of Expertise*. Boston, MA: Mariner Books; 2017.

CHAPTER 2
Learning Goals

Case Study

M.P. is a second-year pharmacy student who is struggling with pharmacokinetics and pharmacology courses. The student is frustrated that despite understanding the material, test grades are not satisfactory. Often helping partners in a study group understand difficult concepts, those friends can't understand why M.P. is doing so poorly in these courses. During one of our meetings, we complete an exam wrapper, a tool for analyzing exam performance, and discover that M.P. is having difficulty remembering basic facts needed to answer questions and is struggling to solve pharmacokinetic problems on tests. The student states that most of the time spent studying is "really trying to understand the concepts being taught in class." M.P. feels that committing the facts and information to memory and attempting practicing problems cannot begin without a full understanding of the course material. The student admits to spending little time doing either of these before the exam.

CASE STUDY ANALYSIS

The barrier this student is facing is a lack of understanding of the learning process and what goals should be achieved while studying. The student's goal of developing an in-depth understanding of the concepts is admirable and certainly necessary for mastery; however, the time spent on achieving this goal leaves little or no time for other equally important goals like encoding, consolidation, and application. This is a problem that I see in many of my students. The key to removing this barrier is an understanding that mastering concepts is a process and requires achievement of four major learning goals. In this chapter we are going to explore those goals and a process that you can use to ensure that you achieve them.

Understanding how we learn is important to maximize learning. Based on educational literature and my experience as both a student and teacher, I have created a very basic model that describes the different learning goals to which you should aspire in the process of content mastery. Keep in mind that learning is a complex process that is significantly more nuanced than what I am about to describe. The four-part learning goals model is loosely based on levels of learning described by Bloom's revised taxonomy of educational objectives and those which occur in the daily life of a typical student.[1] They are designed to provide you with specific targets or milestones that you need to achieve to master a particular concept or subject area. One thing to keep in mind is that learning something new is a process. Acquisition of knowledge does not occur instantly and requires the learner to work to achieve each of the major learning goals. When learning new material, being able to identify what learning goals need to be achieved can help you be a more effective and efficient learner.

Learning Goal 1: Priming for Learning

Preparation for learning is an important step in mastering a concept yet is one that most students will ignore. If you have ever gone to class not knowing what you were going to learn or were lost or wished you had asked an important clarifying question, then you know about what I am talking. The good news is that achieving this goal is simple and should take no more than 20 minutes of your time. This process includes identifying and analyzing learning goals and objectives for class, determining how materials for class are organized, identifying challenging content, and reactivating previously learned and related knowledge. I have found that students who achieve this learning goal have a much more effective classroom experience. They come to class knowing what they are going to learn that day, have reactivated or recalled related knowledge on which to build their learning, they are less likely to get lost during class, and are ready to ask specific and meaningful questions that will help with their learning. For those of you who are enrolled in a program where team- or problem-based learning is used, preclass preparation becomes even more critical for your learning. Not only do you need to have a basic familiarity with the material, but you are expected to come to class with an understanding of the material that will allow you to immediately participate in assessments and class activities involving problem solving. In Chapter 3 you will learn about strategies that can help you to achieve learning goal.[1]

Learning Goal 2: Understanding and Building Context

For students in a lecture-based course, developing a basic understanding of concepts begins in the classroom. When learners arrive to class having already exposed themselves to new material, they are better able to engage in the process of understanding and connecting it to prior knowledge. One of the major mistakes that students with whom I work make is treating class as a passive learning experience. This is especially true if they are taking a lecture-based course. Taking handwritten notes, listening carefully, focusing and thinking about what the instructor is telling you, asking appropriate questions, and working with classmates on active learning exercises are critical to maximizing classroom learning.

For students taking a team- or problem-based learning class, understanding and building context begins outside the classroom and will continue during your class session. In these types of courses, you must engage with the material assigned to you prior to class. A strong understanding of basic concepts and how they relate to one another will help you to successfully navigate individual and team-based assessments as well as to engage in different learning activities.

Building context is an important part of active studying and begins in the classroom. Contextualization of new concepts occurs when you begin to determine how new information is related with information you have already learned. For example, if you are in a pharmacology class learning about the mechanism of action of beta-adrenergic antagonists, you can very quickly build context by relating this class of drugs to knowledge you gained in a prior physiology class on neurotransmission in the sympathetic nervous system and blood pressure regulation.

Learning Goal 3: Memory Formation and Strengthening

Often the most lengthy and critical parts of learning is the formation of a durable working knowledge base through memory formation and strengthening.[2] Achieving this learning goal takes place during studying and involves multiple steps: encoding, consolidation, storage, and reconsolidation. Simply put, encoding is the process of converting sensory information (what you see on your notes, what the instructor is saying) into mental representations. Consolidation and storage involve strengthening these mental representations in long-term memory storage. Reconsolidation is a process that involves repeatedly recalling information to ensure information stays in long-term memory. This process may seem complicated, but you have successfully completed these steps throughout your entire life without even knowing it. The most important aspect of this learning goal is to ensure you allocate enough time to achieve it as memory formation and strengthening take time.

One final thought about this process. Do not confuse it with memorization. While there are some similarities, they are significantly different processes. Memorization does not require understanding, contextualization, or reflection on the part of the learner about what was learned, why it is important, and how it is connected to preexisting knowledge. For example, you can memorize a list of words in a foreign language or a sequence of numbers without knowing what they mean or how to appropriately use them in a sentence. Without meaning, this information is not very useful for achieving the next learning goal, utilization.

Learning Goal 4: Utilization

This final goal of learning is often the most complex and challenging for students but is arguably the most important. While being able to understand and accurately recall theoretical concepts and facts is important, it is not terribly useful unless you can use that information to solve problems on an exam or care for your future patients. I chose the term "utilization" for this final learning goal as I wanted one that would broadly encapsulate all of the higher order learning competencies that students might be expected to achieve.[1] These include application of concepts, analysis and evaluation of information, and creation. Unfortunately, I have found that practicing application of concepts is often one of the last things students do prior to an examination, and at that point it may be too late. Practicing application of material can and should occur as early as step two of the S.A.L.A.M.I. method and continue throughout the consolidation phase. Opportunities for application of information can come in many formats and can be created by the instructor or the student. Application of knowledge is easily the most "active" part of the learning process as it generally required students to take the knowledge and contextual understanding of information that they have gained through the first three steps and use them to problem solve.

Stages of Learning, the S.A.L.A.M.I. Steps, and Content Mastery

Up to this point we have identified the 5 different steps in the S.A.L.A.M.I. method:

1. **Preclass preparation**
2. **In-class engagement**
3. **Postclass review**
4. **Preexam preparation**
5. **Postassessment review**

We have also discussed the 4 learning goals and the differences between them. Now we are going to examine how the steps and learning goals come together to help you achieve content mastery.

Figure 2-1 depicts the relationship between the 4 learning goals and the 5 different steps of the S.A.L.A.M.I. method.

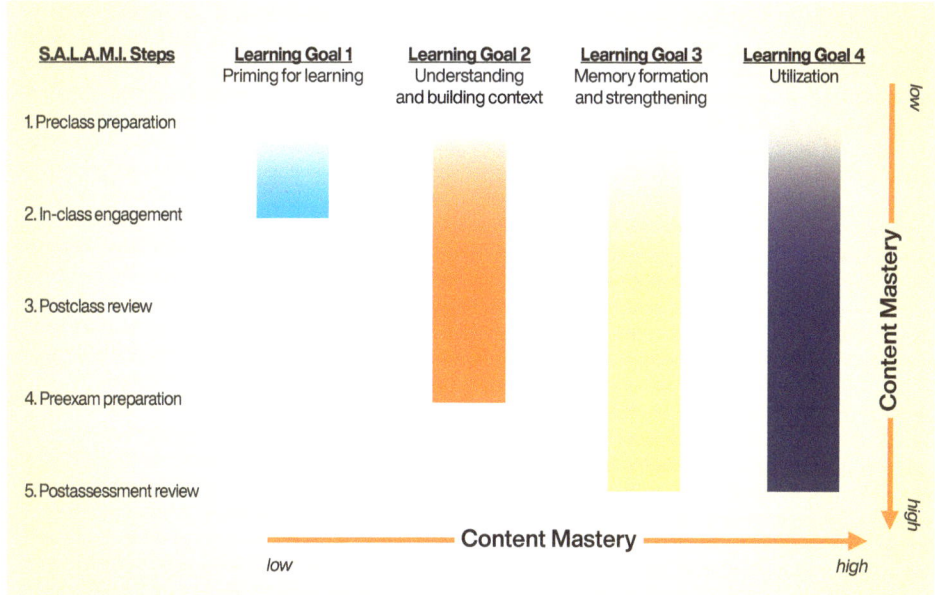

Figure 2-1: Learning Goals and the S.A.L.A.M.I. Method

The above figure represents a very basic model of learning that demonstrates the relationship between the five steps of the S.A.L.A.M.I. method and the four basic learning goals, critical for content mastery. Shaded and colored rectangles represent the importance of achieving each learning goal during a particular step of the S.A.L.A.M.I. method. Darker shading represents a higher importance and lighter shading, the opposite.

Each of the colored rectangles in Figure 2-1 is shaded with a color gradient. The darker the color in the rectangle, the more likely that stage is to be achieved during the corresponding S.A.L.A.M.I. step. For example, the blue rectangle represents learning goal 1, priming for learning. Developing familiarity with material begins while preparing for an upcoming class and should peak either during or directly afterwards. The peak of priming for learning is represented by the darker blue color in the rectangle. While you may be introduced to "new" material after class (concepts you might have missed if you were distracted or sleeping), this should be the exception rather than the rule. The blue rectangle, therefore, ends right after S.A.L.A.M.I. step 2, in-class engagement. Notice that the yellow and green rectangles on the right side of the diagram begin with priming for learning and culminate during preparation for an exam. Keep in mind that this diagram is meant to represent how the learning goals and S.A.L.A.M.I. steps are interconnected. In reality, learning is a lot more complicated and messier!

Monday	Class 1 Material	Priming for learning	+	Understanding	
Tuesday	Class 1 Material	Understanding	+	Memory formation and strengthening	
Wednesday	Class 1 Material	Memory formation and strengthening	+	Utilization	
	Class 2 Material	Priming for learning	+	Understanding	
Thursday	Class 1 Material	Memory formation and strengthening	+	Utilization	
	Class 2 Material	Understanding	+	Memory formation and strengthening	
Friday	Class 1 Material	Memory formation and strengthening	+	Utilization	
	Class 2 Material	Memory formation and strengthening	+	Utilization	
	Class 3 Material	Priming for learning	+	Understanding	

Figure 2-2: Achievement of Learning Goals Through the Week

The figure above is a hypothetical example of how the four-stage model of learning might be used to map out preparation for a three-credit course that meets for one hour on *Monday, Wednesday and Friday*. The color scheme used represents each of the four learning goals. The length of each of the colored rectangles depicts the amount of time or effort spent on achieving each of the learning goals on that day and with that material.

Figure 2-2 is a hypothetical example of how the four learning goals might be achieved through the week. In this example I am using a three-credit course that meets for one hour on Monday, Wednesday, and Friday. The color scheme used represents each of the four learning goals. The length of each of the colored rectangles depicts the amount of time or effort spent on achieving each of the learning goals on that day and with that material. As you review this figure consider how the learning process depicted differs from the one that you are currently using.

One key feature depicted by Figure 2-2 is that the material covered in each of the classes is studied daily. This is one of the most important parts of the S.A.L.A.M.I. method; taking small bites of the material each day so that it can be completely digested over a longer period. Breaking your learning down in this way requires that you are organized, utilize a schedule, employ a wide range of learning techniques, are flexible, consistently measure your level of mastery, and use that information to subsequently shape future learning sessions. You should also note that how you study concepts and your goals for learning change from day to day.

In the following chapters, we will discuss various steps that can be taken to ensure productive learning and begin to explore each of the five steps of the S.A.L.A.M.I. method. Based on my experience as a teacher and academic coach, I have provided specific examples of techniques or strategies that students can use during each of the five steps. Using these strategies will help you get the most out of the different steps of the process and help you to move through the four learning goals more quickly and efficiently.

Key Concepts from Chapter 2

1. In my mental model of learning there are four learning goals that students need to achieve on their way to mastering material. They are priming for learning, understanding and building context, memory formation, and strengthening and utilization.

2. Building a durable, working knowledge base is a process that takes time and involves encoding, consolidation, storage, and reconsolidation.

3. Developing metacognitive knowledge, control, and regulation and using evidence-based learning strategies like active recall, spacing, elaboration, and interleaving are necessary to successfully complete the five steps of the S.A.L.A.M.I. method; preclass preparation, in-class engagement, postclass review, preexam preparation, and postassessment review.

REFERENCES
1. Anderson LW, Krathwohl D. *A Taxonomy for Learning, Teaching, and Assessing: A Revision of Bloom's Taxonomy of Educational Objectives.* Boston, MA: Allyn & Bacon: 2001.
2. Dudai Y. The neurobiology of consolidations, or, how stable is the engram? *Ann RePsychol.* 2004;55:51-86.

CHAPTER 3
Productivity

Case Study

A.L. is a first-year pharmacy student who has failed three out of four exams so far. The student performed well as an undergraduate but tells me of feeling completely overwhelmed by the volume of material that must be learned in such a short period of time. A.L. also tells me of being very distracted while trying to study, preferring to do most of their work at the campus student center. The student drinks five to six large energy drinks every day to stay up late to study, but this results in difficulty falling asleep at night. A.L. has never heard of active recall or spacing and spends a considerable amount of time recopying class notes.

CASE STUDY ANALYSIS

With the rapid pace at which you have to learn large amounts of material, there is no wonder why many pharmacy students feel overwhelmed their first semester of pharmacy school. There is a significant difference in learning expectations in a professional degree program. A.L. is going through what I refer to as the "adjustment period." While every student makes this transition, some make it more quickly than others. Those who transition quickly have either acquired effective learning skills or do so relatively quickly. Those who don't transition quickly may struggle initially like A.L. One of the areas with which students struggle is how to be productive in their learning. If you look at A.L.'s case closely, you might find several things with which you identify with. In this chapter we are going to examine the various components of productivity, what can go wrong, and how you can benefit from the enormous amount of research that has been done in this area to help you be a more effective learner.

Productivity

For many years as a faculty member, I would spend considerable time working with struggling students on time management. I would talk to them about creating a weekly and daily schedule, how to block out time for studying, commuting, sleeping, eating, doing laundry, and exercise and then encourage them to follow it. For some students the act of creating and following a structured schedule was enough to get them moving in the right direction, but for many it wasn't enough. Through the years as I learned more about time management and the behaviors that could derail it, I began to understand that time management was only one small component of being productive as a student.

Productivity is a characteristic with which many people are fascinated. It has been studied and written about extensively. Many of the most popular books like *The 7 Habits of Highly Successful People: Powerful Lessons in Personal Change* and *Getting Things Done: The Art of Stress-Free Productivity* were written by successful business people.[1,2] While the concepts in these books are extremely useful and can be applied to many different settings, I felt that developing a model based on commonly recognized components of productivity for students might be helpful. In this model I included what I think are the nine most important components of academic productivity (Figure 3-1).

1. **Motivation**
2. **Focus**
3. **Process and approach to studying**
4. **Environment**

5. Organization
6. Goal setting and prioritization
7. Preparation
8. Time management
9. Wellness

All these components are discussed throughout the book, however, I am going to highlight several below.

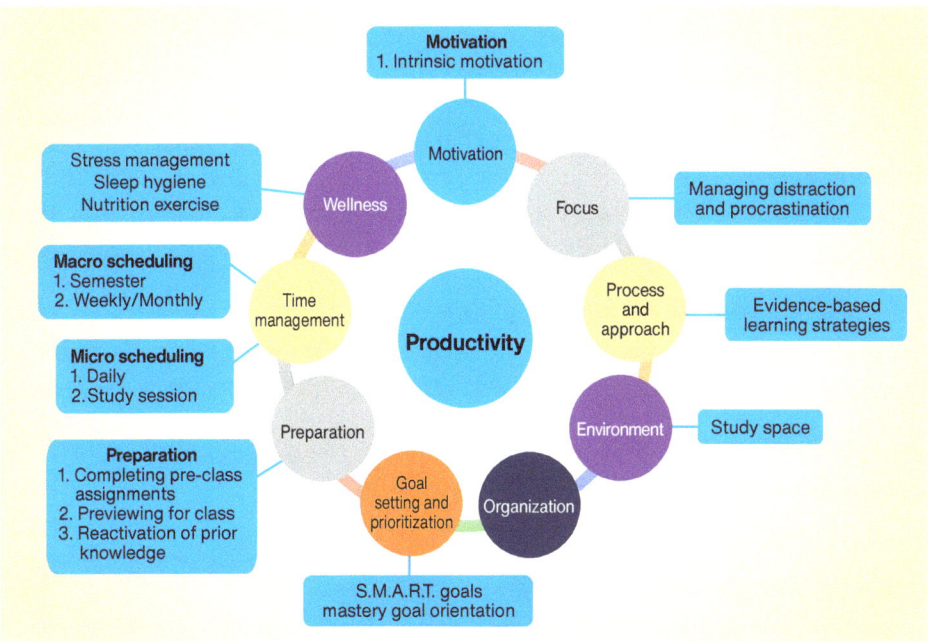

Figure 3-1: Components of Academic Productivity
The nine different components of productivity are all interrelated and are necessary in order to be maximally productive with your learning.

WELLNESS

I should not have to tell you that stress is synonymous with pharmacy school. On any given day you are probably juggling test preparation, meeting project deadlines, completing cocurricular and interprofessional education requirements, introductory pharmacy practice experiences (IPPEs) and advanced pharmacy practice experiences (APPEs), and these are just the things associated with school. The most common types of negative stressors I see with my students that are associated with poor academic performance fall into three general categories: personal issues (end of a relationship, moving, family divorce), financial (student loan debt, paying bills), and health related. Regardless of the source, stress can have a crippling effect on mental and physical health and in turn derail even the best student's academic performance. Excessive stress can have a significant negative impact on pharmacy students and has been extensively studied. A recent study out of the University of California San Diego, Skaggs School of Pharmacy and Pharmaceutical Sciences, showed a worsening of stress, an increase in the use of maladaptive coping strategies, and worsening of mental health affected the quality of life of students as they progressed through preclinical program.[3] Other studies have shown a clear correlation between stress and the performance of the part of memory that is critical for short-term storage and use of information called working memory.[4,5] Working, or short-term (as it is often called), memory is critically important for learning and problem solving.

While it is not within the scope of this book to address each type of stress that a student might experience or to provide specific advice about how to deal with that stress, I do want to emphasize that addressing external stressors is critical. Most college campuses have significant resources and infrastructure in place to help students deal with stress. These include exercise facilities, campus counseling centers, and places to engage in prayer and meditation. Family and friends can be a great source of support, as well as professors, advisors, and student affairs and financial aid staff. Additionally, many campuses offer wellness programs for students. The bottom line is that you should never ignore abnormal stress and hope that it will just go away. Being proactive and leaning into the problems associated with stress is the best way to gain confidence and grow.

Students should never underestimate the importance of wellness in the learning process. In a weeklong workshop that I offer to our first-year pharmacy students to learn evidence-based learning strategies, a significant part of the week is devoted to wellness and wellness activities. Getting appropriate amounts of sleep, exercise, and nutritional food is critical for every stage of the learning process and very much in your control. Unfortunately, when things start to get hectic, these necessities are often the first to be cast aside to make room for course preparation. When this happens, it can have a significant impact on our ability to learn and apply new information. It also indicates that your time management strategy, number of courses you are taking, extracurricular activities, and work schedule needs to be reevaluated.

SLEEP

Sleep deprivation is something with which most students are familiar. Think about your own experience with sleep during the academic year. Do you consistently tend to stay up late at night to study? Do you tend to fall into irregular sleep patterns, staying up all night only to catch a few hours of sleep before morning? If you answered yes to these questions, you are not alone. A study published in the *American*

Journal of Pharmaceutical Education in 2015 reported the sleep habits of 364 Auburn University Pharmacy students. More than half of the students surveyed obtained six or less hours of sleep a night and an even greater number (81.7%) got less than seven hours of sleep the night before an examination. In addition, nearly half of these students experienced daily symptoms of daytime sleepiness. More importantly this study showed a positive correlation between getting enough sleep the night before an examination translated into higher course and semester grades.[6]

Scientific studies have demonstrated that the normal functioning of many bodily processes is highly dependent on the amount of sleep one gets, and sleep deprivation has been associated with changes in the activity of the autonomic nervous, endocrine, and immune systems.[7] Additionally, numerous studies have demonstrated that a lack of sleep can have a negative impact on cognitive performance and memory consolidation.[8,9] Despite the evidence in the medical literature and their own personal experiences, most students will sacrifice sleep, especially as a major exam is approaching to gain, a few extra hours of studying. Because of the significant impact that acute and chronic sleep deprivation can have on cognitive function, these students are doing themselves much more harm than good. In addition, they are depriving themselves of a type of cognitive processing that occurs during periods of restfulness known as the diffuse mode of thinking.

In her book *A Mind for Numbers,* Barbara Oakley describes how the brain can switch between and use different "modes of thinking" by engaging different neural networks. These networks are associated with either the highly attentive or "focused mode" of thinking or the more "relaxed resting state networks" referred to as the diffuse mode of thinking. The focused mode of thinking is associated with the prefrontal cortex in the brain and concentration. It appears to be engaged and used during activities like direct problem solving. The diffuse mode of thinking appears to be an unconscious process that is always "on in the background." It can play a significant role in processing information associated with a problem or concepts with which you might be struggling. Have you ever been stuck on a complex math problem and walked away from it for a short period, only to come back to it and discover the solution was right in front of your nose? That's the diffuse mode, and its importance in information processing and problem solving should not be underestimated.[10]

ENVIRONMENT

What makes a productive study space? This is one of the most critical questions to ask and answer before using the S.A.L.A.M.I. method. I believe that a productive study space should meet the following criteria:

1. It should be comfortable (but not too comfortable).
2. It should be safe.
3. It should be free of clutter.
4. It should be easily accessible.
5. It should be free of distraction.

The following is a description of the pros and cons of four commonly used study spaces. These locations along with my generalizations and judgments are based on my own experiences and discussions with hundreds of students over many years. Your experience with these spaces may vary depending on your individual circumstances and preferences.

Residence

A person's place of residence, such as a dorm room, apartment, or house, is one of the most common and convenient choices for a study space. One of its primary benefits being convenience. Generally, it is the most accessible study space and eliminates the need to travel to a different area once you return from classes. In this space, you have the most control over your environment. You can design and create your own study space. You can adjust the lighting and temperature to suit your preferences. You have easy access to amenities like food, restroom facilities, and, hopefully, the space is safe. There are also downsides to studying where you live. If you share your living space with someone, that person can unknowingly serve as a major barrier to your study efforts. Roommates, who are not academically focused or motivated, can often weaken the resolve of any student who is determined to study. The added activity and noise generated by a roommate, whether on a computer, watching TV, eating, or sleeping can be a major barrier to a focused study session. Parents and loved ones, despite their best intentions, can be a huge distraction especially if you are living with them while you are in school. Housekeeping chores like cleaning the bathroom, doing laundry, or cleaning out your closet or junk drawer might seem like a preferable option to hitting the books. The temptation to sleep (especially if your study space is in your bedroom), talk to someone, go online, or be distracted by some other activity is also high.

Library

The campus library is also a common place for students to study. Campus libraries are typically very accessible, have optimal environmental conditions for study, and most likely have key informational resources that can help with research or gain clarity on a difficult topic. In addition, many library spaces have private study rooms, cubicles, or cubbies that can help cut down on potential distractions. The key to deciding whether the library will be a productive study environment is to identify how many potential distractors you might encounter. The most common complaint about the library that

I hear from students involve interruptions by classmates looking for a study break or asking a question about class material. These seemingly innocent visits can easily turn into 45-minute conversations that interrupt the rhythm and focus you need for productive studying. To avoid these issues, a local public or collegiate library that is not frequented by fellow classmates can be an excellent alternative.

Public Spaces

Although the idea of sitting in a comfortable chair, sipping on a nice cup of coffee at your local coffee shop while studying for your upcoming pharmacokinetics examination sounds wonderful, it may not be conducive for productive learning. Your working memory only has a limited capacity to process and store information and can be overwhelmed by the excessive audio, visual, olfactory, and gustatory distractions in this environment. These can interfere with focus and interrupt opportunities for productive study. As an avid coffee drinker, my advice is go to your local cafe, but get your cup of coffee to go!

Campus Classrooms

Empty campus classrooms, if accessible after hours, can be an excellent place to study. The functional design of campus classrooms and environmental conditions provide a nice balance between comfort and productivity, and, I know from firsthand experience, it is hard (but not impossible) to fall asleep at a classroom desk. Studying in campus classrooms make a lot of sense if you live on campus or stay after your last class of the day and your college or university allows it. Classrooms are typically uncluttered and free from many types of distractions. Furthermore, many of your fellow classmates, after a long day of classes, want nothing more than to escape the building they have been in all day and get home. This can work to your advantage and can cut down on many of the distractions you might encounter in other locations.

Safety on a college campus varies from institution to institution and is a very important consideration when choosing a study space. Some important questions to ask yourself about studying in an empty classroom study space, especially after normal business hours include

1. **How many people are in the building in which you are studying?**
2. **Does campus security have a strong presence in that building?**
3. **Is it safe to walk to your car or other forms of transportation after dark?**

In order to focus and concentrate, it is important to know and feel that you are safe. Anything less than that can be a powerful distractor and keep you from achieving the four learning goals.

There are many study-space options available to students. Ultimately it is up to the individual to make a judgment on what space will work best. My best advice is that when looking for a study space, use the five criteria above to gauge how productive your space will likely be.

When I discuss the issue of study space with students, inevitably someone asks whether one should study in one or more locations? The answer to that depends on several factors. Let's briefly consider some of the work that has been done in this area. Most of such research suggests that our ability to encode information is strongly linked to our emotional and physical state as well as the environmental cues we experience when we are learning. Much of the research suggests that introducing variety into the way that we study, such as using different active recall techniques, interleaving different subjects, or even changing the environment in which we study can introduce what is referred to as desirable difficulties. These positive barriers to learning seem to enhance our ability to encode and recall information from our long-term memory. We know that the brain depends heavily on emotional, physical, and environmental cues to access information successfully from long-term memory and that attempts to recall information, whether successful or not, significantly improves the ability to recall that information later.[11,12] An important study in this area by Smith, Glenberg and Bjork in 1978 demonstrated that recall of information after multiple study sessions was higher in participants that studied in multiple locations. It was suggested that a change in environmental cues while learning (i.e., the study environment) might have a positive impact on the brains ability to recall.[13] In a second study, Smith and Rothkopf had two groups of students watch statistics lectures either in one room or in four different rooms and tested retention of information five days later. The group that watched the lectures in the four different rooms was able to retain more information than the group that watched the lecture in only one.[14] These studies suggest that if you study and practice recall in multiple locations throughout the day, you may be able to improve your retention of information. One thing to keep in mind is that if you use multiple areas for study, make sure that they meet the criteria laid out above. Any gains you might make in long-term retention of information by studying in multiple locations could be easily offset by distractors or safety issues inherent in one of those spaces.

TIME MANAGEMENT

There is a whole industry dedicated to teaching people good time-management strategies. Everything from books to YouTube videos to workshops and many apps are available to help us manage this precious resource, yet there is very little research directing us on what techniques, skills, and approaches are the most effective. As such, I offer a few insights and what I consider to be best practices in this area.

Most of my students who display characteristics of effective time management keep two distinct calendars. One calendar shows all their major deadlines, assignment due dates, and examinations over the course of the semester. Many have this calendar displayed over their study area where it provides a big picture view of upcoming assignment due dates, examinations, work schedule, and co- and extracurricular events. The second is a more detailed calendar that displays daily activities, which allows them to plan out effectively their studying throughout the day. I have seen students use paper daily planners, Excel spreadsheets, and calendar functions in Microsoft Office or Google. They all seem to work equally well. Your choice of what to use should be based on what is easiest for you to use. If your calendar isn't easily accessible throughout the day, it is unlikely that you will use it to make strategic decisions about how to allocate your time. Personally, I have been using the calendar in Outlook for years to manage my schedule. I like that it allows me to look at my schedule from several different perspectives. I can get a "bird's eye view" of major events and deadlines over a several month period, or I can zoom in to track what is going on every 30 minutes during my day. As a bonus, I have access to it on my work laptop and cell phone which means I can access it whenever I need to. I can also set up reminders for upcoming events and deadlines.

Many of you might balk at living a life dictated by a planner or calendar. You might argue that schedules are difficult to follow and that they don't allow for the flexibility to respond to unseen events. Both arguments have merit; however, I believe the benefits of following some sort of calendar significantly outweigh the detriments. Prior to setting up your long-range and daily calendar, I encourage you to map out what a typical week in school looks like for you. This map can be created in Excel, on paper, or in a table created in Microsoft Word. It can be extremely useful in helping you quickly identify where your free time is so that you can use that time more effectively. This map can also be helpful as you begin to lay out your two calendars.

Figure 3-2 is a "map" of what a "typical" first-year pharmacy student's first semester might look like. This "map" was made with Excel, includes only classes and labs, and uses a color coding scheme that quickly allows you to identify free time, as well as important and reoccurring events. Class and labs are represented by different colors, and the white space represents free time. In this version of the map there is quite a bit of free time between 6:00 AM and 11:00 PM throughout the week. This free time can be used to accomplish personal tasks, to study, to complete assignments, to engage in self-care, and to schedule outside work with employers.

Time	Monday	Tuesday	Wednesday	Thursday	Friday	Saturday	Sunday
6:00							
6:30							
7:00							
7:30							
8:00		Anatomy and physiology		Anatomy and physiology			
8:30	Biochemistry	Anatomy and physiology	Biochemistry	Anatomy and physiology			
9:00							
9:30					Embedded IPPE experiences or school events		
10:00					Embedded IPPE experiences or school events		
10:30					Embedded IPPE experiences or school events		
11:00		Dean's hour		Team-based/ Co-curricular Activities/Review Sessions/Meetings		
11:30	Pharmaceutics I lecture	Dean's hour	Pharmaceutics I lecture	Team-based/ Co-curricular Activities/Review Sessions/Meetings		
12:00	Pharmaceutics I lecture		Pharmaceutics I lecture	Team-based/ Co-curricular Activities/Review Sessions/Meetings		
12:30		University activity hour					
1:00		University activity hour					
1:30							
2:00		Pharmaceutical calculations		Pharmaceutical calculations			
2:30		Pharmaceutical calculations		Pharmaceutical calculations			
3:00	Pharmaceutics lab	Elective course	Pharmacy skills laboratory	Elective course	Anatomy and physiology laboratory		
3:30	Pharmaceutics lab	Elective course	Pharmacy skills laboratory	Elective course	Anatomy and physiology laboratory		
4:00							
4:30							
5:00							
5:30							
6:00							
6:30							
7:00							
7:30							
8:00							
8:30							
9:00							
9:30							
10:00							
10:30							
11:00							

Figure 3-2: Example of a First-Year Pharmacy Student's Weekly Schedule
The figure above is a hypothetical schedule for a first-year pharmacy student. Classes and weekly activities are color coded for quick identification. Free time is noted by white space.

Once your class schedule is filled in on your map, the next step is to identify blocks of time that can be used for studying. When scheduling time to study you have four different options. These include studying before, in-between and after classes, as well as on the weekend. Of these four, most students tend to schedule the bulk of their study time after-class, especially later in the evening. The advantage of studying at this time is that the concepts you learned in class that day are freshest in your mind. Studying after classes also gives you an opportunity to engage in postclass review. This activity is discussed in Chapter 6 and provides you with an important opportunity to evaluate your basic level of understanding of concepts and to begin the encoding process. There are several downsides to studying after classes end. The first is that it may be difficult to get motivated to study once you have returned home and had a chance to relax. Additionally, many students will study late into the night, experiencing greatly diminished returns on their effort as it gets later and later. If you are one of these students, I would like to recommend that you complete your studying before midnight. This will give you a chance to unwind after a long day and maximize the amount of sleep that you are likely to get.

   I have also worked with students that enjoy getting up early and studying before their classes begin in the morning. This can be a great time to be productive. The early mornings tend to be very quiet and free of distraction, especially if you are on campus. The downside, of course, is that if you are already fatigued, it can be difficult to get out of bed early in the morning. A third option includes studying in-between classes. Many students fail to take advantage of the time that they have in-between classes. You would be surprised at what you can achieve in a 20- to 30-minute window, especially if you use high impact study strategies like active recall. Even on very busy days, piecing together two to three hours of studying from breaks in-between classes is possible.

   Finally, the weekend is an important time to clean up any areas of confusion, to practice application, and to continue to reinforce concepts that you have learned throughout the week. The key to productive weekends is your schedule. Plan and mark your calendars with the times that you plan on studying and stick to them. Do not study more than three to four hours without at least an hour break afterwards. Many students who study on the weekend choose to engage in long, marathon study sessions. These sessions tend to be very unproductive as most people lose focus and drive after a few hours. So why do students choose this approach? For many, sitting and studying for six, eight, or more hours makes them feel productive; however, the actual amount of work that they accomplished is often much less than they think. If you are someone that studies on the weekends in this way, take a minute and really think about how productive you are. How many times are you distracted? How many breaks do you take? Are you using low-impact study strategies like rereading or recopying your notes or listening to lectures again in their entirety? If you answered yes to any of these questions, I would encourage you to take a different approach. Instead of one, long marathon session, divide it up. Study for three to four hours in the morning and then reengage later in the afternoon. This allows for a significant buffer in between sessions that will give your brain a chance to rest and process information, and you will have an opportunity to engage in other activities.

A common question that I get from new students is, "How much time should I study during the week." A common rule of thumb indicates that for every hour of class you should spend two to three hours studying outside of class. While I think this is a good place to start, it can be difficult for students to conceptualize what this means and how to achieve it. I use a slightly different approach by comparing student academic loads with a 40-hour work week. Most student academic loads run between 17 to 20 credit hours per semester which translates into roughly 17 to 20 hours of class time per week. With this in mind, I encourage my students to commit to an additional 20+ hours of work outside of class to do the equivalent work associated with a 40-hour work week. If this sounds like a lot to you, remember that most adults live relatively normal and happy lives working this much during the week and many work a lot more! In fact, if you think about how much your peers in the workforce are working, many are pulling 50- to 60-hour work weeks as they begin to establish themselves in their respective careers.

If you have never spent 20 hours a week studying, achieving this goal can seem nearly impossible, but it isn't. The maps (Figure 3-2 and 3-3) are key to making this happen. For you to achieve the goal of studying 20 hours per week will simply require some minor additions. Take a few minutes to think about all of the daily, non-school related activities (i.e., eating, sleeping, laundry, commuting, exercise, grocery shopping, etc.) and begin to enter them onto your schedule. After that has been completed, your schedule may look something like Figure 3-3.

CHAPTER 3 - PRODUCTIVITY

Time	Monday	Tuesday	Wednesday	Thursday	Friday	Saturday	Sunday
6:00	Wake-up exercise, get ready, drive to school	Wake-up exercise, get ready, drive to school	Wake-up exercise, get ready, drive to school	Wake-up exercise, get ready, drive to school	Wake-up exercise, get ready, drive to school		
6:30							
7:00							
7:30							
8:00	Biochemistry	Anatomy and physiology	Biochemistry	Anatomy and physiology			
8:30							
9:00							
9:30	Break	Break	Break	Break	Embedded IPPE experiences or school events		Breakfast laundry, grocery shopping
10:00	Study	Study	Study	Study			
10:30							
11:00	Pharmaceutics I lecture	Dean's hour	Pharmaceutics I lecture	Team-based/ Co-curricular Activities/Review Sessions/Meetings			
11:30							
12:00		Break					
12:30		University activity hour					Lunch
1:00	Lunch		Lunch	Lunch	Lunch		
1:30		Break					
2:00	Pharmaceutics lab	Pharmaceutical calculations	Pharmacy skills laboratory	Pharmaceutical calculations	Anatomy and physiology laboratory	Work	Study
2:30							
3:00		Elective course		Elective course			
3:30							
4:00							
4:30		Study		Study			
5:00					Break		
5:30	Dinner and break		Dinner and break				Dinner and break
6:00							
6:30		Dinner and break		Dinner and break			
7:00					Work		
7:30							
8:00	Study	Study	Study	Study			Study
8:30							
9:00							
9:30							
10:00							
10:30							
11:00							

Figure 3-3: Example of a First-Year Pharmacy Student's Weekly Schedule

The figure above is a hypothetical schedule for a first-year pharmacy student. Classes and weekly activities are color coded for quick identification. In this schedule, time for personal activities like eating, exercise, and commute times are added in. Free time is noted by white space.

As you can see from this hypothetical calendar, some of the initial white space in Figure 3-2 has been replaced by 20 hours of red study blocks, daily life activities (yellow), and work (purple). In addition, there are blocked times during the day for a university activity hour, team-based and cocurricular activities, and IPPEs that may not be needed every week, thus giving you even more free time.

Once you have your calendar completed, it is time to take it for a "test drive" to see how realistic it is. When setting up your schedule for the week, you may have over- or underestimated the time it will take to complete certain activities. You may have also forgotten to include important activities in your schedule. Careful monitoring of how well you can follow your schedule while making appropriate changes is critical for effective time management. For example, you may find that after two weeks of following your schedule you just can't seem to sit down for that Wednesday evening study session. You might need to alter your schedule to accommodate this study time, move this study block to another section of your schedule, or come up with a strategy that will help you avoid the Wednesday night distractors that are keeping you from studying. Keep in mind that the schedule that you initially come up with will most likely change over time. There is nothing wrong with this if the changes do not impede your ability to achieve the four learning goals. My recommendation is that for the first month or so, you should evaluate how well you follow your schedule on a weekly basis and make any necessary changes. Once you feel comfortable that the schedule meets your needs, a weekly review is no longer needed unless major changes in your class or personal schedule are imminent.

FOCUS

As with deliberate practice, the S.A.L.A.M.I. method is most successful when the student is completely focused. A number of studies have shown that distractions from a variety of sources impair learning both in and out of the classroom.[15,16] In fact, certain types of distractions have been shown to impair our ability to judge how well we have learned something. To fully understand both the time one needs to allocate for learning and the importance of minimizing distraction while studying, a brief discussion of human memory is necessary.

While our understanding of memory is continually evolving, most neuroscientists working in the field of human cognition believe that human beings possess multiple types of memory. These include short-term, working, and long-term memory.[17] Short-term memory temporarily holds small amounts of information for short periods of time.[18,19] Working memory, which is closely associated with short-term memory, is believed to be important in reasoning and decision making and is associated with problem solving.[20] Long-term memory is the part of memory where facts and information are stored for long periods of time.[19] One of your primary goals while studying is to successfully store information with a high degree of fidelity into long-term memory, where it can be accessed later to solve examination problems or care for a patient. Visual and auditory information captured while studying is processed by short-term and working memory before it is encoded into long-term memory. Studies suggest that the amount of information that can be handled by working memory at any given time is extremely finite, with estimates of four to seven "slots" available for information storage.[21]

A number of studies suggest that auditory distractions and using multiple forms of media can have negative impacts on short-term and working memory.[22-24] When we allow these types of distractors into our study sessions, we are handicapping ourselves by allowing them to interfere with our learning. Apparently, the amount of learning that can be achieved in the presence of a distraction might be dependent on the study method you are using. A study by Buchin and Mulligan demonstrated that the memory encoding effects associated with using retrieval practice are much more resistant to the negative effects of distraction than just reviewing your class notes.[25] The bottom line of eliminating distractions while you study is always better; but, if there are some that are outside of your control, using retrieval practice may help to eliminate their negative effects.

When I was a student, my primary distractors were the phone in my apartment, my television, and my bed. Because of these distractions, I did most of my studying at the Health Sciences Center in an unused laboratory space. Physical separation from these distractors allowed me the opportunity to really focus on my studies. Unfortunately, because of the portability of today's technology, escaping distractors like social media, streaming video content, and instant communication with friends and family is much more difficult. I consider myself extremely fortunate to have gone to college and graduate school before cell phones, the Internet, and social media. I often laugh and tell my students that I would have failed out of school if I had to contend with the types of distractions associated with modern technology.

Take a moment and think about what distracts you during study. I'd be willing to bet that at the top of your list is your smart phone. Other common distractors with which my students struggle include laptops/tablets, pets, and other human beings. Technology, for better and worse, has transformed the way we learn. It has given us unprecedented access to information at a speed I never could have dreamed of as a graduate student. It allows us to communicate with anyone, anywhere. If used appropriately, technology can enhance the way we learn; however, it can also be a major distraction. If your smart phone is a distractor for you, turn the phone off and put it in a place where you can't see it. Tell family or friends where you are studying in case they need to get a hold of you in an emergency, and only check your phone during planned study breaks.

MOTIVATION

Let's face it. Most students would agree that studying does not make their top ten list of favorite things to do. While studying can be satisfying, especially when you feel you have accomplished something, it is still work. Finding the inspiration necessary to study for hours and adapting a new approach to studying and learning can be difficult. This is where motivation becomes important. Motivation plays an important role in all aspects of our lives, from getting out of bed in the morning, to eating healthy and exercising, to working on a project or studying. It turns out that what motivates you may have an important impact on learning.[26] Take a moment and think about what motivates you to study. Is it an interest in the subject you are studying? Are you motivated by good grades? Do you believe that learning about a subject can help with future job performance? Does your motivation come from a fear of failure or a belief that it is what you are supposed to do as a student?

Numerous studies support the finding that the type of motivation can have a significant impact on learning. There are three basic types of motivation referenced in the literature: intrinsic, extrinsic, and amotivation.[27] Students who are intrinsically motivated to learn might choose to study because they are interested in learning about a topic or derive self-satisfaction or pleasure from doing so. Students who are externally motivated might study because they believe it will help make them a better practitioner, they want to earn a specific grade, they feel pressure to study from peers, parents, or instructors, or they are simply afraid of failing. Students who are amotivated tend not to study. They believe that they have little control of their academic success and that no matter what they do, they will only get bad grades.[28] I have seen students influenced by each of these types of motivators, and I believe that if you can change your motivation from an amotivation mindset to an intrinsically motivated one, learning becomes more enjoyable, less stressful, and, as a result, you become more successful.

Daniel Pink, author of *Drive*, spoke about the "Puzzle of Motivation" during a TED Talk® he gave in 2009 (www.ted.com/talks/dan_pink_the_puzzle_of_motivation). As a business analyst, his perspective on motivation centers around job performance; however, I believe that his ideas about motivation can be effectively applied to studying and learning and the educational literature backs me up on this. In his talk, Pink argues that "contingent or extrinsic motivators" (rewards for high performance) subdues creativity and productivity. This practice has been used extensively in business to motivate workers using pay raises and bonuses. While this strategy does increase productivity in mindless, repetitive tasks, it decreases performance on tasks requiring some level of cognitive processing and creativity. He then sites psychological and sociologic studies that verify this relationship. It seems to me that there might be an important connections between the phenomena that Pink is describing and the type of motivation you experience and the type of study technique you might choose to use.

Many of the students with whom I work come into pharmacy school having done well in their undergraduate studies by using a cramming or "massed practice" method of studying. This method involves mindless, repetitive drilling of information usually right before an exam. Many earned good grades, minimizing the work they needed to do outside of class. Unfortunately, the cost of this approach is typically a minimal understanding of concepts and poor long-term retention of information. After beginning their first semester of pharmacy school and performing poorly on initial assessments, they realize that this strategy is not going to work. Having nothing left to fall back on, they become discouraged and amotivated. This can be a significant issue because there seems to be a positive correlation between motivation and metacognition that can have a significant impact on academic success.[29] Students who are amotivated can struggle significantly leading to a further decline in learning and grades, which can quickly become a serious academic issue. While these types of study techniques have been shown to promote short-term retention of information, they do not promote long-term retention.

Intrinsically motivated students tend to be more effective learners than those who are motivated by external factors.[30] These types of students are in pharmacy school because they want to pursue a career that is meaningful to them. They find the information that they learn is interesting and relevant to their career goals. When they inevitably encounter subjects that are dry or uninteresting, they can use their internal motivation to help maintain their learning and motivation in these classes. Their intrinsic locus of motivation may predispose them to look for ways to connect what they are currently learning to prior and future learning. Making these types of mental connections, especially between prior and new knowledge is a powerful way to learn and to retain information.[31]

Your motivation to study and learn can be influenced by your perceived competence in a subject area and the amount of autonomy you have over your own learning.[26] I have worked with students who have performed poorly on assessments and feel as though they have little control over their own learning. These students are at risk of becoming amotivated. Once they begin to develop and implement an effective study plan and to meet their own internal expectations for exam performance, their motivation begins to shift. Part of my own academic transformation that occurred in graduate school was due to a shift in my motivation and my belief that I could learn more effectively. Like many undergraduates, I was very grade-focused and had a healthy fear of academic failure. Even though I knew it was important to learn and had possessed some degree of interest in my studies, my primary motivation was to pass my classes. In graduate school my motivation to study and learn shifted from a fear and goal orientation to one focused on personal and professional growth. I learned and studied because I enjoyed the material and truly believed it was important component of my training as a scientist. This shift occurred for two major reasons. I was engaged in a field of study in which I was interested and the study methodology I learned from the physiology teaching team gave me a sense of autonomy and control over my learning. As my confidence grew from having a structured study strategy, my anxiety and fear of not performing well academically was significantly reduced.

How can you change your orientation from being a type-A or externally motivated student to one who relies on intrinsic motivation? In his TED Talk® Pink identifies three major components of intrinsic motivation: autonomy, mastery and purpose. One of the major benefits of the S.A.L.A.M.I. method is that it will give you more autonomy and self-regulation over your learning. Successful, self-regulated learners differ from other learners in that they have an awareness of how they learn best, have the skills necessary to achieve learning goals independently, understand when they have achieved those goals, and can adapt to a variety of learning environments and academic challenges.[32] The S.A.L.A.M.I. method will give you the tools to become a self-regulated learner who is motivated and equipped to initiate the learning process on your own, to set goals for learning, identify and employ appropriate strategies to learn and evaluate how successful you are at learning. It does this by (1) providing you with a structured approach to learning that can be applied to a variety of academic settings, (2) teaching you how to gauge and monitor the level of mastery of a subject so that gaps in knowledge can be filled, and (3) providing you with the knowledge of evidence-based learning strategies and how to implement them in your study. Once you realize that you have control over learning, your motivation to learn can change and you can become less dependent on what is going on in the classroom. This is particularly important when less-than-optimal teaching and learning approaches are being used by an instructor. When employed correctly, the S.A.L.A.M.I method can help with mastery of knowledge.

Key Concepts from Chapter 3

1. **Physical, mental, and emotional stress can have a significant impact on your learning. Being mindful of the types of stressors you are experiencing and seeking out appropriate support are important considerations.**

2. **Finding a good study space is critically important. Wherever you study, ensure that the following criteria are met:**
    - **Appropriate level of comfort (but not too comfortable)**
    - **Safety**
    - **Free of clutter**
    - **Easily accessible**
    - **FREE OF DISTRACTION**

3. Academic productivity has six different components: motivation, process and approach, organization, goal setting and prioritization, preparation, and time management. Maximizing these six components will help you to become a more effective and efficient learner.

4. Mapping out daily activities and developing a schedule can reveal free time during your day that you can use for studying. It can also help you use this free time more effectively.

REFERENCES

1. Covey SR, Covey S. *The 7 Habits of Highly Effective People: Powerful Lessons in Personal Change*. New York, NY: Simon & Schuster; 2020.
2. Allen D. *Getting Things Done: The Art of Stress-Free Productivity*. Revised edition. New York, NY: Penguin Books; 2015.
3. Hirsch JD, Nemlekar P, Phuong P, et al. Patterns of stress, coping and health-related quality of life in doctor of pharmacy students. *Am J Pharm Educ*. 2020;84(3):7547. doi:10.5688/ajpe7547.
4. Luethi M. Stress effects on working memory, explicit memory, and implicit memory for neutral and emotional stimuli in healthy men. *Front Behav Neurosci*. 2008;2. doi:10.3389/neuro.08.005.2008.
5. Yuan Y, Leung AWS, Duan H, et al. The effects of long-term stress on neural dynamics of working memory processing: an investigation using ERP. *Sci Rep*. 2016;6(1):23217. doi:10.1038/srep23217.
6. Zeek ML, Savoie MJ, Song M, et al. Sleep duration and academic performance among student pharmacists. *Am J Pharm Educ*. 2015;79(5):63. doi:10.5688/ajpe79563.
7. Alhoa P, Polo-Kantola P. Sleep deprivation: impact on cognitive performance. *Neuropsychiatr Treat*. 2007;3(5):553-567.
8. Maquet P. The role of sleep in learning and memory. *Science*. 2001;294(5544):1048-1052. doi:10.1126/science.1062856.
9. Stickgold R. Sleep-dependent memory consolidation. *Nature*. 2005;437(7063):1272-1278. doi:10.1038/nature04286.
10. Oakley B. *A Mind for Numbers: How to Excel at Math and Science (Even If You Flunked Algebra)*. New York, NY: Jeremy P. Tarcher/Penguin; 2014.
11. Bjork, RA. Memory and metamemory considerations in the training of human beings. In: Metcalfe J, Shimamura AP, eds. *Metacognition*. Cambridge, MA: The MIT Press; 1994:185-205. doi:10.7551/mitpress/4561.003.0011.
12. Bjork EL, Bjork RA. Making things hard on yourself, but in a good way: creating desirable difficulties to enhance learning. In: Gernsbacher E, Pew RW, Hough LM, Pomerantz JR, eds. *Psychology and the Real World: Essays Illustrating Fundamental Contributions to Society*. New York, NY: Worth Publishers; 2011:56-64.
13. Smith SM, Glenberg A, Bjork RA. Environmental context and human memory. *Mem Cognit*. 1978;6(4):342-353.
14. Smith S, Rothkopf E. Contextual enrichment and distribution of practice in the classroom. *Cogn Instr*. 1984;1(3):341-358.
15. Glass AL, Kang M. Dividing attention in the classroom reduces exam performance. *Educ Psychol*. 2019;39(3):395-408. doi:10.1080/01443410.2018.1489046.

16. Blasiman RN, Larabee D, Fabry D. Distracted students: a comparison of multiple types of distractions on learning in online lectures. *Scholarsh Teach Learn Psychol*. 2018;4(4):222-230. doi:10.1037/stl0000122.
17. Cowan N. What are the differences between long-term, short-term, and working memory? In: Sossin WS, Lacaille J-C, Castellucci VF, Belleville S, eds. *Progress in Brain Research*. Vol 169. Amsterdam, The Netherlands: Elsevier; 2008:323-338. doi:10.1016/S0079-6123(07)00020-9.
18. Broadbent DE. *Perception and Communication*. Oxford, England: Pergamon Press; 1958. doi:10.1037/10037-000.
19. Atkinson RC, Shiffrin RM. Human memory: a proposed system and its control processes. In: Spence KW, Spence JT, eds. *Psychology of Learning and Motivation*. Vol 2. Amsterdam, The Netherlands: Elsevier; 1968:89-195. doi:10.1016/S0079-7421(08)60422-3.
20. Miller GA, Galanter E, Pribram KH, eds. *Plans and the structure of behavior*. New York, NY: Henry Holt and Company; 1960. doi:10.1002/cne.901150208.
21. Miller GA. The magical number seven, plus or minus two: some limits on our capacity for processing information. *Psychol Rev*. 1994;101(2):343-352. doi:10.1037/0033-295X.101.2.343.
22. Uncapher MR, Thieu MK, Wagner AD. Media multitasking and memory: differences in working memory and long-term memory. *Psychon Bull Rev*. 2016;23(2):483-490. doi:10.3758/s13423-015-0907-3.
23. Hughes RW, Marsh JE. When is forewarned forearmed? Predicting auditory distraction in short-term memory. *J Exp Psychol Learn Mem Cogn*. 2020;46(3):427-442. doi:10.1037/xlm0000736.
24. Banbury SP, Macken WJ, Tremblay S, Jones DM. Auditory distraction and short-term memory: phenomena and practical implications. *Hum Factors J Hum Factors Ergon Soc*. 2001;43(1):12-29. doi:10.1518/001872001775992462.
25. Buchin ZL, Mulligan NW. Divided attention and the encoding effects of retrieval. *Q J Exp Psychol*. 2019;72(10):2474-2494. doi:10.1177/1747021819847141.
26. Schunk DH. Self-efficacy and academic motivation. *Educ Psychol*. 1991;26:207-223.
27. Ryan RM, Deci EL. Intrinsic and extrinsic motivations: classic definitions and new directions. *Contemp Educ Psychol*. 2000;25(1):54-67. doi:10.1006/ceps.1999.1020.
28. Deci EL, Vallerand RJ, Pelletier LG, Ryan RM. Motivation and education: the self-determination perspective. *Educ Psychol*. 1991;26(3-4):325-346.
29. Landine J, Stewart J. Relationship between metacognition, motivation, locus of control, self-efficacy, and academic achievement. *Can J Couns*. 1998;32(3):200-212.
30. Vallerand RJ, Pelletier LG, Blais MR, Briere NM, Senecal C, Vallieres EF. The academic motivation scale: a measure of intrinsic, extrinsic, and amotivation in education. *Educ Psychol Meas*. 1992;52(4):1003-1017. doi:10.1177/0013164492052004025.
31. Bransford JD, ed. *How People Learn: Brain, Mind, Experience, and School: Expanded Edition*. Washington, DC: National Academies Press; 2000. doi:10.17226/9853.
32. Bjork RA, Dunlosky J, Kornell N. Self-regulated learning: beliefs, techniques, and illusions. *Annu Rev Psychol*. 2013;64(1):417-444. doi:10.1146/annurev-psych-113011-143823.

CHAPTER 4
S.A.L.A.M.I. Method Step 1: Preclass Preparation

Case Study

B.R. is a third-year pharmacy student who is performing poorly in a cardiovascular disease course that I teach. The student came to me for help concerned that even with spending an excessive amount of time studying for my course, grades continued to remain poor. I asked about the student's approach to studying. B.R. would listen to the day's lecture at least twice before studying the class notes. When asked to explain the rationale for that strategy, the student admitted to never knowing what the instructor was going to cover each day and learning very little from class. B.R.'s mind often wandered, resulting in being lost and remembering very little about what was taught in class.

CASE STUDY ANALYSIS

B.R.'s challenge is one that I see often. Despite good intentions, many students do not get the learning benefit that they can out of class because they do nothing to prepare for it beforehand. As a result, they are often lost, frustrated, and demotivated and end up doing a lot of catch-up work afterwards. In this chapter we discuss strategies that will help you get more out of your class experience before you even go to class.

The primary goal of the S.A.L.A.M.I. method step 1 is "priming" your brain for learning. This is done before class to help you identify the main topics that will be covered and to analyze the lecture's objectives. By reactivating relevant prior knowledge and beginning to build familiarity with new concepts, you are setting yourself up for success. There are several priming strategies that you can use to accomplish these goals. Some are as simple as performing a simple analysis of lecture notes or slides, completing preassigned readings, or watching an online video on the subject material. In fact, many successful students use a combination of these approaches as a way of preparing for their next class. Like me, they have found that the 10-15 minutes spent preparing for the following day's lecture can make a significant difference in how much they get out of class the next day.

Previewing

Some of you reading this text might recall a time when GPS was not available to the public. If you were going on a trip, you consulted Rand-McNally, picked up a TripTik at AAA, or consulted some type of online website like MapQuest to generate directions to your destination. In those days, planning your trip was the key to avoiding anxiety and stress as well as to maximizing your enjoyment. Just taking a few minutes to review the route before leaving could help avoid missing important turn-offs, finding key spots to stop, and preventing getting hopelessly lost. The idea of pre-planning to maximize your trip experience can be readily applied to studying. This strategy is commonly referred to as previewing.

When I was first introduced to the concept of previewing in graduate school, it was presented as a quick, simple, and efficient way to become familiar with new material. Despite its simplicity, I found it to be transformative for my learning. What I love about previewing is that when done correctly you get a significant boost in your learning for a small investment in time. The main goal of previewing is to prepare for learning during the next day's class. Using the analogy above, the notes given to you by your instructors are your "road map" and previewing is "a way to familiarize yourself with the map and plot out your course" before starting class.

Before previewing new material, there are several "rules" with which to be familiar.

1. Previewing new class material should take no more than 10-20 minutes.

2. Previewing can be applied to note packets, PowerPoint® presentations, assigned readings, or other learning materials.

3. Your goal for previewing is to build *familiarity and context* and begin to reactivate prior knowledge related to concepts being introduced the next day.

4. Previewing does not involve memorization or attempting to develop a deep understanding or mastery of the material. Remember we are just reviewing our "directions" for tomorrow's "trip" to have a better understanding of where we are headed, what to watch out for, and when not to fall asleep or mentally wander off!

To start the process of previewing, asking yourself five key questions about the concepts you are about to learn is helpful.

1. What will I be learning and why is it important?

2. What do I already know about this material?

3. What are the learning objectives or goals for class, and how do they inform me about learning expectations?

4. What is new or looks confusing in the notes or reading assignment?

5. What resources are available to help with my learning?

From these five questions, I have developed a simple learning tool that you can use to guide yourself through the previewing process. This tool is available for free with the digital version of the book on PharmacyLibrary.com. Let's look at each of these questions and why they are important to consider.

WHAT WILL I BE LEARNING AND WHY IS IT IMPORTANT?

In most cases, identifying the major concepts covered in each class should not be difficult. At a minimum, this information should be specified in the course syllabus under the schedule of topics. Additionally, most note packets or PowerPoint slides have a title page or section and preassigned lecture notes and slides. Assigned readings can also provide additional "clues" to what topics you will be learning in an upcoming class.

Reflecting on the importance of what you are learning is an important part of developing metacognitive awareness. It always surprises me how many students with whom I work don't fully understand the rationale behind what they are learning. They struggle to see how new material is relevant and valuable to their professional development and view certain types of learning as busy work or certain courses as hurdles that simply need to be overcome so they can get a degree. This type of thinking only promotes the type of surface learning that we are trying to avoid with the S.A.L.A.M.I. method. As I reflect on my time as an undergraduate, I see how painfully obvious much of my own academic struggle was directly related to this type of thinking. This all changed when I went to graduate school and the interconnection between what I was learning and my own research became clear. Each class I attended provided me with a new piece to a much larger puzzle. What also became very clear was how much I learned and how well I learned it would have a lasting impact on my career.

WHAT DO I ALREADY KNOW ABOUT THIS MATERIAL? (REACTIVATING PRIOR KNOWLEDGE)

Learning new information is easier when it can be related to prior knowledge,[1] and the positive benefits of reactivating prior knowledge to learning new skills has been well documented.[2-4] Most academic programs, including pharmacy, provide instruction in foundational areas first and then cover more complex, specific, and advanced content that build on that foundation. For example, most pharmacy students are required to take courses in anatomy, physiology, biochemistry, microbiology, and immunology either as prerequisites or in the first year of their programs. The concepts taught in these courses form a critical foundation for the understanding of more specific and focused practice-related disciplines like pathophysiology, pharmacology, or therapeutics. To effectively master these more advanced subjects, using our preexisting knowledge as a foundation for learning is important. During previewing, you can repurpose a common classroom active learning strategy called focused listing to aid in this process.

When used in previewing, focused listing relies on a reactivation of knowledge strategy called mobilization. Mobilization requires you to bring to mind all prior knowledge about a particular topic you are trying to learn.[5] Let's say you are previewing a lecture on breast cancer for an oncology course. Chances are you have some prior knowledge of this topic, whether it was taught in a formal academic setting or learned from other sources. To use the focused listing technique, brainstorm a list of a few simple facts or terms that you can remember related to breast cancer. Hopefully some of these facts will come from prior coursework but can also come from other sources as well. Your list might look something like this.

Breast Cancer

1. Genetic causes: HER2, brc1. (I remember this from my biochemistry course.)
2. Environmental causes: smoking, hormone replacement therapy. (I heard this on the news.)
3. Menopause. (I think this might be related somehow.)
4. Tamoxifen. (I'm not sure what it does.)
5. Classification by different stages. (My aunt had stage 2 breast cancer.)
6. Estrogen (I learned about this hormone in physiology class.)
7. Metastasis (I read about this in a magazine article on cancer.)

In addition to listing facts, you should also try to remember where or how you learned them. Generating these lists should not take more than several minutes. During this exercise, you should not be looking up information online or referencing old course material. The level of detail and factual correctness at this stage is not important, rather "activating" any prior knowledge on the topic by attempting to remember it is the goal. By activating prior knowledge of a topic, you are beginning the process of building context and reconstructing information from long term memory.[6] This will help you more fully to understand new information being taught in class. Once you are in class or directly after, compare your list with what you learned. Ask yourself what is missing, what is incorrect, or what misconceptions about the topic you had that are now altered by what you learned in class. Focus listing can also be used in S.A.L.A.M.I. steps 3 and 4 to help in the process of building context, increasing understanding, and facilitating consolidation.

WHAT ARE THE LEARNING OBJECTIVES OR GOALS FOR CLASS?

The next step in previewing is to identify and analyze the primary learning goals for the next day's class. Most faculty communicate these expectations through learning objectives that are presented at the beginning of lectures or classroom activities and can be found in accompanying PowerPoint presentations and handouts. Skilled instructors will begin to develop class materials by creating learning objectives based on Bloom's Taxonomy of Learning.[7] Bloom's Taxonomy of Learning is an extremely useful classification scheme that allows faculty members to communicate expectations for student learning through their course and lecture learning objectives. Bloom's taxonomy is divided into six distinct hierarchical categories: remember, understand, apply, analyze, evaluate, and create. The category to which each of the learning objectives belongs can be determined by the "Bloom's verbs" that are found at the beginning of most learning objectives.

Learning objectives optimally serve as a framework that faculty use for developing content for a class and for determining the type of instructional strategies and assessments to be used. As such, learning how to deconstruct and analyze learning objectives is a great way to "crack open" a lecture. Good learning objectives reflect the major concepts and skills that the instructors want their students to know and have, which is why it is important for you to pay careful attention to them. For example, if an instructor uses verbs in an objectives like "list," "define," and "identify," you can reasonably assume that the expectation for learning will be based largely on being able to remember information. If verbs such as "explain," "describe," "compare," and "contrast" are used, the level of learning required is understanding. If, however, verbs like "create," "justify," "assess," "derive," "construct," "determine" are used, this implies that higher order thinking, applying, analyzing, evaluating, and creating both in class and on assessment are necessary.

Let's practice analyzing learning objectives by using a set from a pharmacology lecture on receptor and dose-response theory.

1. **Describe** drug-receptor interactions using the **law of mass** action.

2. **Derive** the formula for **binding affinity (K_d)** from the law of mass action.

3. **Construct** and **analyze** a **dose-response curve** from raw data to include the proper labeling of the x- and y-axis, **ED_{50}**, **threshold value**, and **E_{max}**.

4. **Explain** how **potency** and **efficacy** are represented on a dose-response curve.

5. **Determine** the potency and **intrinsic activity** of a drug from dose-response curves.

6. **Explain** the relationship between ED_{50} and binding affinity

What important information can be gained from these objectives? Based on the verbs used in these objectives ("derive," "construct," "analyze," and "determine") some higher order thinking and application of concepts will be required. There are several objectives that use verbs ("describe," "explain") implying that remembering and recalling information will be important. In addition, specific terminology (highlighted in blue in the list above) can provide clues about important concepts that should be learned during this class period. These highlighted terms can also be helpful when using the focused listing exercise to help identify and reactivate prior knowledge.

Unfortunately, some faculty do not use learning objectives in their courses. If you find yourself in this situation, there are several steps you can take that might help. Taking a few minutes to scan your book or class materials can help determine what topics will be taught. If you are assigned readings from a textbook, you are likely to find a group of learning objectives at the beginning of each chapter. If you are assigned practice problems, read through them quickly and try to determine their level of difficulty. Do the problems require you to simply remember and understand information, or do they require you to apply what you have learned in more complex ways? This quick analysis can give you some insight into your instructor's expectations for learning.

When you have familiarized yourself with the learning objectives, you will have a better understanding of what you will be learning in your upcoming class and what the instructor's expectations are for thinking about the material. Learning objectives are also useful when you are studying and preparing for an upcoming assessment, and I will show you how they can be used effectively for this purpose in upcoming chapters.

WHAT IS NEW OR LOOKS CONFUSING IN THE NOTES OR READING ASSIGNMENT?

The next step in the previewing process is scanning your notes or slides for unfamiliar concepts, terms, and figures, graphs, or tables that might be important to understand. Below are 3 pages from a hypothetical pharmacology/medicinal chemistry handout on diabetes. Take a few minutes and scan the following pages. Identify the main concepts covered by these pages. Circle or highlight terms and concepts with which you are unfamiliar. Mark any figures or diagrams that you might be confusing or unfamiliar.

Secretagogues

I. Sulfonylureas

    A. Medicinal Chemistry
       General Information

            a) Divided into 2 groups or generations: first- and second-generation analogues

General Chemical Structure

R_1—⟨benzene⟩—SO_2NHCNH—R_2 (with C=O)

b) All members of this class of drugs are substituted arylsulfonylureas

c) Differ by substitutions at the R1 para position on the benzene ring and at the R2 nitrogen residue of the urea moiety

d) First-generation agents characterized by small R1 substituents: CH3, Cl, COOH

e) Second-generation agents developed for

(1) Increased potency

(2) More rapid onset of action

(3) Longer duration of action

(4) Shorter plasma t1/2

II. Second-Generation Sulfonylureas

A. Contain ρ-(β-aryl carboxy amido ethyl) Group

1. Increases binding affinity to target protein

2. Biggest difference between first- and second-generation drugs

Glyburide (Micronase®, Diabeta®, Glynase®)

Glipizide (Glucotrol®)

B. Normal Physiologic Activity of β cells (see figure of pancreatic β cell below)

1. **Step 1.** Increase in plasma glucose (i.e., after a meal)

2. **Step 2.** Elevated plasma glucose levels causes an increase in β cell uptake of glucose (via GLUT2 transporter protein)

3. **Step 3.** Glucose molecules undergo glycolysis (via TCA cycle) producing ATP

4. **Step 4.** ATP binds to Kir6.2 subunit causing ATP-sensitive K+ channels to close

5. **Step 5.** Thus, positively charged K+ ions build up on the inside of the cell membrane causing it to depolarize. This depolarization triggers voltage-gated calcium channels to open

6. **Step 6.** The resulting elevation of intracellular calcium levels triggers an increase in the release of insulin into the blood stream

Pancreatic β Cell

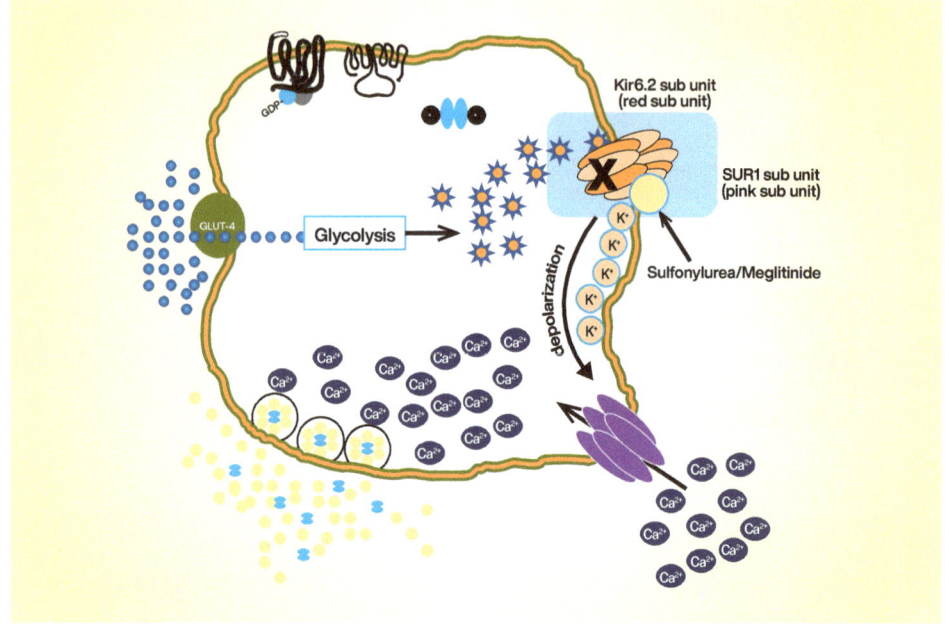

C. Mechanism of Action

    1. Effects of Sulfonylureas on Insulin Release

        a. Sulfonylureas bind to SUR1 subunit of ATP sensitive K+ channels in pancreatic β cells **causing the channel to close.**

        b. Subsequent ***depolarization*** of β-cell membranes

        c. Voltage gated Ca^{2+} channels open resulting in an influx of extracellular Ca^{2+}

        d. Ca^{2+} triggers release of insulin from granules

D. Adverse Reactions

    1. Hypoglycemia as a result of oversecretion of insulin

    2. Weight gain as a result of effects of excess insulin on adipose tissue

3. Headache

4. Dizziness

5. Mild gastrointestinal (GI) discomfort

6. Rash and skin reactions

What did you come up with? Perhaps the picture of the pancreatic β-cell caught your attention. Maybe you were unfamiliar with the term "secretagogue." Perhaps you circled or marked the chemical structures knowing that medicinal chemistry is a topic with which you struggle. Each person will inevitably identify different pieces of information based on each's prior knowledge base, familiarity with different topics, or experience with the material. Regardless of what you marked, having specific road marks identified in your notes can help you to pay attention at key moments during class. It may also prompt you to ask questions or do additional research on a subject.

WHAT RESOURCES ARE AVAILABLE TO HELP WITH MY LEARNING?

Identifying available learning resources is critically important for class preparation. Instructors will often provide students with handouts, slides, reading assignments from a textbook or article, instructional videos, or podcasts. The Internet can also supply an endless source of information on any subject. In many cases, the issue for students is not a lack of resources but rather deciding which learning resources are appropriate. I offer several pieces of advice to navigate the sea of learning materials available.

1. Focus on the learning materials that the instructor recommends or provides. These learning materials have been vetted by the instructor for appropriateness and accuracy and are likely a primary source of questions on assessments. Once these materials have been mastered, beginning to evaluate, vet, and learn from other sources such as online tutorials is much easier.

2. Check the credentials of those who develop online learning materials. Ask yourself if they have the expertise necessary to teach you what you need to know. Peer-reviewed resources are often the most reliable and have already been vetted by experts in the field.

3. When in doubt about the accuracy or appropriateness of an online resource, ask your instructor.

The following is a tool that I have created to help students with the previewing process. The components of the tool are described in the text above. An electronic copy of this tool is available for free with the digital version of the book on PharmacyLibrary.com.

Preview Guide Sheet

Class: _____ Date: _____

Instructions: Using available learning materials (notes, slides, readings) for the next day, work through the 5 steps below. This process should take no more than 10-15 minutes.

1. Identify major topics you will be learning and why you think they are important?

2. List any prior or related knowledge about this material. Make sure to verify and validate the completeness and correctness of your list after class.

3. Read through the learning objectives or goals, and identify key words that provide you with insight into the expectations for learning and thinking.

4. Identify and list new or confusing concepts in the notes or reading assignment.

5. Identify and list resources that are available to help with your learning.

Key Concepts from Chapter 4

1. The preclass preparation step of the S.A.L.A.M.I. method should take no more than 10-20 minutes and will help you achieve Learning Goal 1: Priming for Learning.

2. The goal of preclass preparation is to reactivate prior knowledge associated with what you will be learning, to build familiarity and context with concepts being introduced, to determine learning expectations, and to identify areas of potential difficulties.

3. Preclass preparation does not involve memorization or attempting to develop a deep understanding or mastery of the material.

4. To start the process of previewing, ask yourself 5 key questions about the concepts you are about to learn:

    a. What will I be learning and why is it important?

    b. What do I already know about this material?

    c. What are the learning objectives or goals for class?

    d. What is new or looks confusing in the notes or reading assignment?

    e. What resources are available to help with my learning?

REFERENCES

1. Bransford JD, Johnson MK. Contextual prerequisites for understanding: some investigations of comprehension and recall. *J Verbal Learn Verbal Behav*. 1972;11(6):717-726. doi:10.1016/S0022-5371(72)80006-9.

2. Chi MTH, De Leeuw N, Chiu MH, Lavancher C. Eliciting self-explanations improves understanding. *Cogn Sci*. 1994;18(3):439-477. doi:10.1207/s15516709cog1803_3.

3. de Grave WS, Schmidt HG, Boshuizen HP. Effects of problem-based discussion on studying a subsequent text: a randomized trial among first year medical students. *Instr Sci*. 2001;29:33-44.

4. Machiels-Bongaerts M, Schmidt HG, Boshuizen HP, Machiels-Bongaerts M, Schmidt HG, Boshuizen HPA (1995). The effect of prior knowledge activation on text recall: an investigation of two conflicting hypotheses. *Br J Educ Psychol*. 1995;(65):409-423.

5. Peeck J. Effects of mobilization of prior knowledge on free recall. *J Exp Psychol Learn Mem Cogn*. 1982;8(6):608-612.

6. van Kesteren MTR, Krabbendam L, Meeter M. Integrating educational knowledge: reactivation of prior knowledge during educational learning enhances memory integration. *Npj Sci Learn*. 2018;3(1):11. doi:10.1038/s41539-018-0027-8.

7. Anderson LW, Krathwohl D. *A Taxonomy for Learning, Teaching, and Assessing: A Revision of Bloom's Taxonomy of Educational Objectives*. Boston, MA: Allyn & Bacon; 2001.

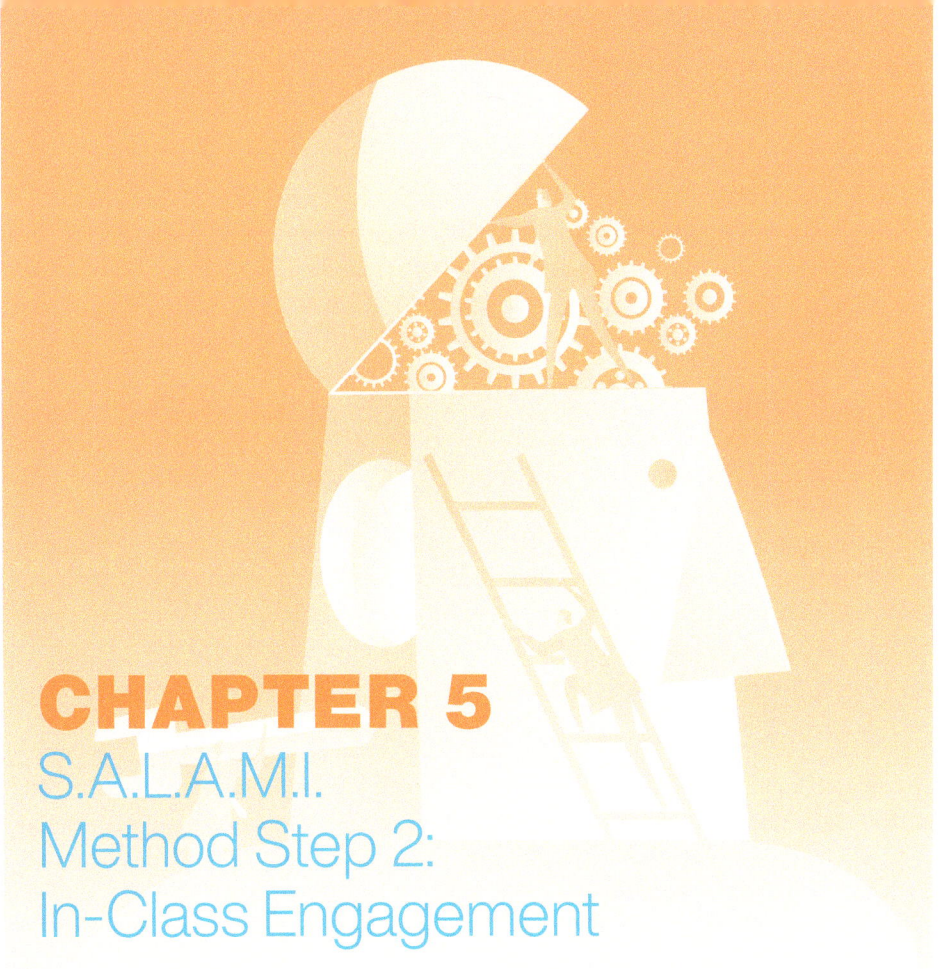

CHAPTER 5
S.A.L.A.M.I. Method Step 2: In-Class Engagement

Case Study

P.N. is a second-year pharmacy student who is struggling in pharmacokinetics and medicinal chemistry courses. During one of our academic coaching meetings, the student reveals that "despite going to class regularly, I don't learn anything and am often lost." P.N. also admits to feeling pressured to have to write down every word the professor says and often comes out of class not knowing what was taught that day. To compensate, P.N. regularly watches lecture recordings, which leave little time to study each night.

CASE STUDY ANALYSIS

Just like P.N., many students I coach have difficulty establishing a strong understanding of complex materials taught during class and, as a result, spend excessive amounts of time outside of class reviewing notes and lecture recordings just to get caught up. These students tend to fall behind quickly and lose valuable time that could be used more efficiently by early engagement of evidence-based learning strategies like active recall.[1] There are at least two reasons that could explain why P.N. is often lost and feels that attending class is a waste of time. First, P.N. may not be effectively preparing for upcoming classes. In the last chapter, you learned about previewing and how it can help you get more out of your classroom learning. The second reason could be attributed to poor note-taking skills. The goal of writing down every word the instructor says during class is unachievable, unproductive, and unnecessary. In this chapter I will teach you how to make informed decisions about whether you need to take notes and, if so, how much. Additionally, you will learn some basic tips for making your note-taking more effective.

The Class Experience

The classroom experience is a valuable opportunity to begin to achieve our second learning goal, understanding and building context. In my experience, however, many students undervalue in-class learning. I believe this is partly due to three issues. The first is that many students lack the skills and strategies needed to learn effectively in class. One of these skills, effective note-taking, is rarely taught despite evidence that suggests it enhances student learning.[2-4] The second is that faculty, and I include myself in this group, do not always use the many pedagogical skills, techniques, and technologies available to fully engage their students in learning. Thirdly, lecture capture technology is readily obtainable and relatively inexpensive, making the availability of high-fidelity lecture recordings more commonplace. As a result, many students believe that class is a waste of time and that they could do just as well in the course skipping class and watching the lecture recording later.[5] In fact, there seems to be a trend in health professions programs, including pharmacy; a sharp decline in class attendance occurs when recorded video lectures are made available to students.[6,7]

This is concerning as numerous studies have demonstrated a positive correlation between classroom attendance and positive academic performance.[8-10] A 2020 research study conducted by Ta and colleagues out of the Washington State University, College of Pharmacy and Pharmaceutical Sciences, looking at the attendance of second-year students in an active learning-based pharmacotherapy course, found a significant negative correlation between students who missed class and their final course grades.[11] In another study, Schnee and colleagues at the Massachusetts College of Pharmacy and Health Sciences looked at the impact of attending live classes versus viewing prerecorded lectures on examination performance in a second-year pharmacy therapeutics course. The authors also found that pharmacy students who attended live classes performed significantly better on exams than those that did not attend a live class.[12] Why is this? Students who go to class can better engage with their instructors about the material being taught. They have opportunities to ask questions and receive answers in a timely fashion. They also have the advantage of participating in important problem-solving and active-learning activities. These activities are designed by instructors to provide their students with the opportunity to practice application of important facts and concepts. In fact, many faculty will model exam questions after active learning exercises and practice problems that they assign. Participation in active-learning exercises is especially important when the instructor is using a flipped classroom model where students develop an understanding of the material outside of class and must come prepared to engage in active learning. Finally, attending class is important for developing the attitudes and skills necessary to be a successful pharmacist.[13,14] Many classes and laboratories in pharmacy school are designed in part to help you learn the professional standards for behavior and practice that you will need to know after you graduate. Furthermore, getting to know your classmates is extremely important. They can be a valuable support network for you during difficult times, and they will become a significant part of your professional network in the future.

Note-Taking

When I was an undergraduate back in the late 80s and early 90s, I relied heavily on note-taking for my learning. All of my classes required me to take extensive notes without the benefit of prepared handouts or slides from which to study. I would sit in class, listen to the professors talk, try to copy the writing on the chalkboard or overhead projector all while trying to make sense of what they were trying to teach me. In fact, I still have some of those notebooks and looking back on them made me realize that I was truly a horrible note taker. I can't begin to imagine how much my learning must have suffered for it! While the methods and technology for note-taking in the classroom have changed significantly since my college days, the habits and motivations for student note-taking have stayed relatively consistent.[15]

There are a number of studies that have been conducted showing the benefit of note-taking to learning.[16,17] While researching this book, however, I quickly began to recognize that the relationship between the two was more complicated and nuanced than I anticipated.[18] In the next section we will take a critical look at the results of some of the more recent studies on note-taking and how these studies can help improve your learning in and out of the classroom.

Purpose of Note-Taking

Researchers have uncovered two benefits of note-taking: creating a durable, written record of what was taught in class, referred to as external storage, and promoting memory formation.[19] Unfortunately, like the evidence-based learning strategies that I teach, most students have never received formal instruction on how or when to take notes which puts them at a significant disadvantage when learning. Like me, the ability of these students to achieve these two goals and to ultimately learn may be lacking. Let's take a closer look at the two benefits associated with note-taking, why each is important, and strategies you can use to achieve them.

External storage of information, the first benefit of note-taking, is achieved when you listen to what your instructor says and record it in a handwritten or typed format. Unfortunately, novice note-takers, especially in situations where the instructor teaches very quickly, can struggle with making rapid decisions about what information needs to be recorded and then accurately capturing it in an organized fashion. One of the most common questions I get about note-taking is whether it is better to handwrite your notes or to type them. As with many of life's important questions, the answer is complicated. There are studies that support the use of both types of note-taking strategies, and, after examining the research in this area, I have made the following conclusions.[20,21] In most cases the way that you take your notes (i.e., written vs. typed) will make little difference in how well you learn provided you abide by the following recommendations. First, reducing distractions while note-taking (especially when using a laptop or tablet) is critical. This means turning off apps, silencing your cell phone, and paying attention in class. Secondly, the process of deciding what information to record and how to summarize or paraphrase it seems to enhance initial memory formation. This means that you shouldn't take mindless dictation during class. Take the time to observe how your instructors teach and learn about their methods of assessment. Before class, analyze the types of learning materials they provide and, most importantly, familiarize yourself with their expectations for learning by examining their learning objectives. For example, if your instructors provide detailed handouts or PowerPoint® slides, or if they tend to read right from their slides, this is a good indicator that the materials provided probably contain most of the important information that you need to learn. In this case, you may not have to take detailed notes and can effectively use handwritten notes that paraphrase or summarize main points so that you can spend more time listening to what is being taught. On the other hand, you might have instructors who provide very sparse learning materials or use a teaching style or pedagogical approach that will require more extensive note-taking. They may teach without the aid of detailed slides or handouts and pause occasionally to write main points on a white- or chalkboard. They may use a flipped classroom model of teaching, where you may be required to read a textbook, paper, or other written materials, watch instructional videos, and take notes to prepare for individual or group-based readiness assessments and problem-solving and application-based learning exercises in class. In each scenario, the notes that you take are likely to be much more extensive and critical for organizing and recording main concepts and important facts and to engage in active recall outside of class. As such, typing your notes on a laptop or tablet may be more beneficial. Finally, don't forget that no matter how you take notes, it's most likely what you do with those notes afterwards that will have the biggest impact on your learning.[15] We will talk in-depth about this in Chapter 7.

The second benefit of note-taking, if it is done correctly, is associated with memory formation. In the field of cognitive psychology, this is often referred to as the encoding effect.[19] Encoding involves the initial transfer of information into memory. This important first step of memory formation is critical to being able to store that information and then recall it accurately and quickly in the future. When students engage in a deeper level of cognitive processing such as making decisions about what information is going to be recorded and how to paraphrase and summarize information, memory formation, i.e., encoding, can be enhanced.[18] Two of the biggest mistakes my students make with note-taking is that they either take no notes or try to record every word the instructor says. Neither approach is very effective at stimulating memory formation because neither allows the opportunity for the learner to begin processing what they are hearing at a deeper level. For example, when students don't take notes, they can easily fall into passive listening, which does not facilitate encoding. Conversely, the cognitive energy that is required for taking dictation does not allow time for the deep processing of information associated with memory formation. I find that in most cases a happy medium can be achieved by listening carefully, making decisions about what information to record, and then paraphrasing or summarizing that information in a written format.

Let's take a moment to examine a picture provided to me by one of my students of notes that taken during several of my cardiovascular lectures (Figure 5-1). The student who took these notes did several things well. Information was accurately captured and successfully paraphrased or summarized in the student's own words. On the other hand, there is a lack of organization or structure in the notes that might make them difficult for studying in the future. Additionally, most of the information recorded on these pages can be found in my handouts and PowerPoint® slides, making much of what was recorded unnecessary.

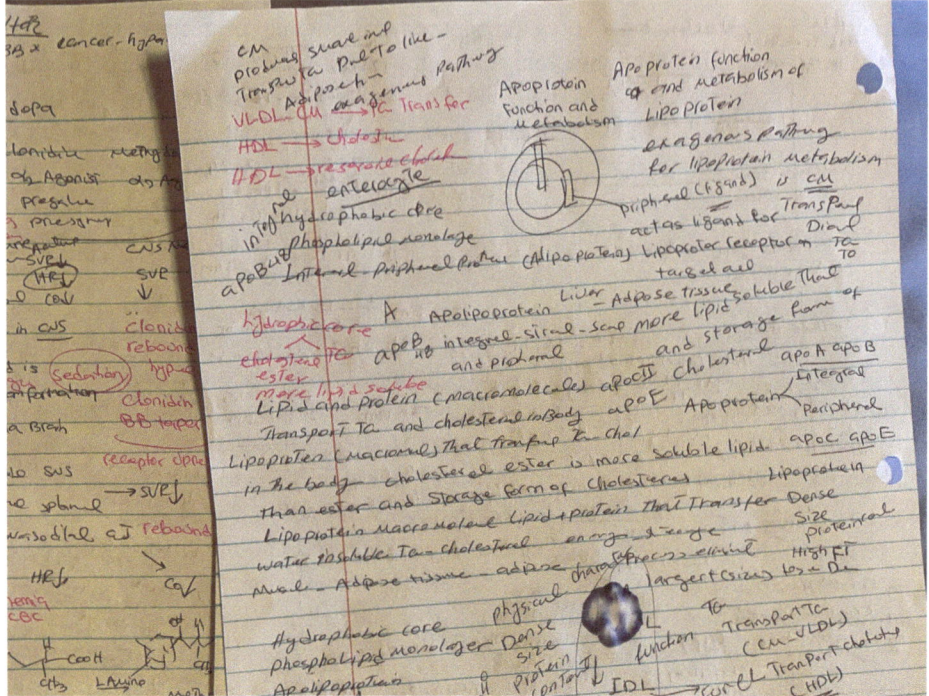

Figure 5-1: Example of Detailed Notes

This is a photo of notes taken by one of my students during lectures I presented on hypertension and hyperlipidemia. At the beginning of the course, I provide students with both the class PowerPoint® Slides and a detailed handout containing most of the information students will need to learn. In this case, it is not necessary for students to take detailed notes, which can free them up to listen, paraphrase and summarize major points that I am teaching. If, however, these types of materials were not provided, then a student would need to take these types of notes.

Note-Taking: When and How Much?

Deciding when and how many notes to take can be difficult as there are so many variables to be considered when making these decisions, including: (1) the type of knowledge that is being taught in class; (2) the type, quality, and density of learning materials that are provided to help guide note-taking (slides or handouts); (3) the amount of mental effort placed on the student during class as they attempt to juggle understanding and processing information they are seeing and hearing with accurate recording of information; and (4) the sources of information the instructor tests from (what is said in class vs. what can be found in a textbook or prepared class notes or slides).

Current educational theory describes four different types of knowledge domains. These include factual, conceptual, procedural, and metacognitive.[22] Courses throughout pharmacy curricula are designed to expose you to each of these types of knowledge; however, from a note-taking standpoint the three on which I am going to focus are factual, conceptual, and procedural. Simply put, factual knowledge is individual pieces of information that can easily be memorized even without context or understanding. Common examples of factual knowledge learned in pharmacy school include drug names, doses, side effects, drug-drug interactions, types of bacteria, genes associated with type 2 diabetes, and lists of different types of protein receptors. If this type of information is available on slides and handouts that your instructor provides, then little note-taking may be required. Conceptual knowledge is generally considered to be more abstract and involves understanding the relationships between separate facts. Examples of conceptual knowledge include learning why certain drugs are categorized as antihypertensive medications, understanding why a specific group of proteins make up a cellular signaling cascade, or why certain type of drugs are administered parenterally and others are administered orally. When instructors are teaching conceptual knowledge, they may use illustrations, graphs, analogies, or examples to describe and explain concepts. In these circumstances, more notes will typically need to be taken to accurately record the analogies, explanations of graphs or diagrams, and real-life examples for future study. Procedural knowledge refers to how to use factual and conceptual knowledge for evaluative and analytical purposes. Examples of procedural knowledge include recommending an appropriate medication for a patient, compounding a medication into a specific dosage form, or solving a pharmacokinetics problem. This type of knowledge is usually gained through a combination of explanation, active learning, and hands-on application. Some notes may be needed in this case but in my experience, engaging and participating in whatever activity is being used for learning is more important rather than trying to capture information for future study. Because many classes you take will involve acquisition of all four types of knowledge, you will likely have to quickly adjust your note-taking according to the type of knowledge you are being taught.

The type of learning materials provided for use in class (handouts, slides, etc.) can also have a significant impact on the choice to take notes and how you take them. Variables to consider when making this decision are the type of knowledge, the amount, and the density of information contained within the learning materials. To illustrate how these variables can have an impact on your note-taking, let's look at three different PowerPoint® slides that I use in class to teach blood pressure regulation.

Type and Density of Knowledge and Note-Taking

EXAMPLE 1. FACTUAL KNOWLEDGE

In example 1, we have a slide (Figure 5-2) that contains exclusively factual knowledge and is very complete with regard to information. My expectations for learning from this slide are that students simply remember the three major factors that have an impact on total peripheral resistance. If the students had previewed the night before, they would know that in subsequent slides I would explain these three factors in more detail. In this example, no notes need to be taken and the student can practice active recall right from the slide when studying.

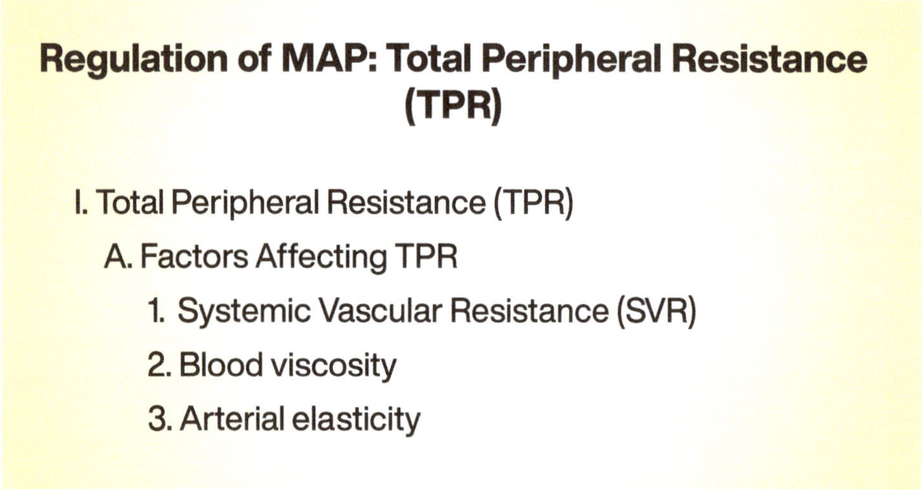

Regulation of MAP: Total Peripheral Resistance (TPR)

I. Total Peripheral Resistance (TPR)
   A. Factors Affecting TPR
      1. Systemic Vascular Resistance (SVR)
      2. Blood viscosity
      3. Arterial elasticity

Figure 5-2: Slide Requiring Little to No Note-Taking

This slide from a blood pressure regulation class that I teach contains factual knowledge and the information on the slide is complete. Students listening to me teach from this slide should not have to take any notes.

EXAMPLE 2: FACTUAL AND CONCEPTUAL KNOWLEDGE

In the slide (Figure 5-3) for example 2, I am teaching both factual and conceptual knowledge, which will require more note-taking than in example 1. The factual knowledge listed on the slide includes the four factors that can have an impact on preload. The conceptual knowledge deals with how those four factors (venous return, capacity, blood volume, and afterload) must change to increase preload and how that, in turn, will increase cardiac contractility. Students may find that they must take more notes on this slide to record my explanation of the diagram and the analogy used to explain how changing preload can affect cardiac contractility.

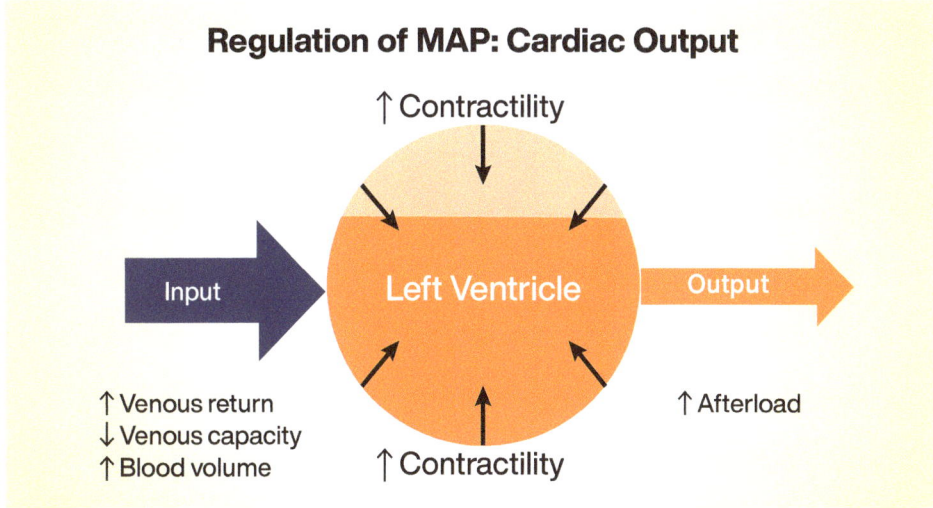

Figure 5-3: Slide Requiring Some Note-Taking

This slide from a blood pressure regulation class that I teach contains both factual and conceptual knowledge. Students may need to take notes on my explanation of this figure or the analogy that I use to explain the impact of preload on cardiac contractility.

EXAMPLE 3: COGNITIVE LOAD

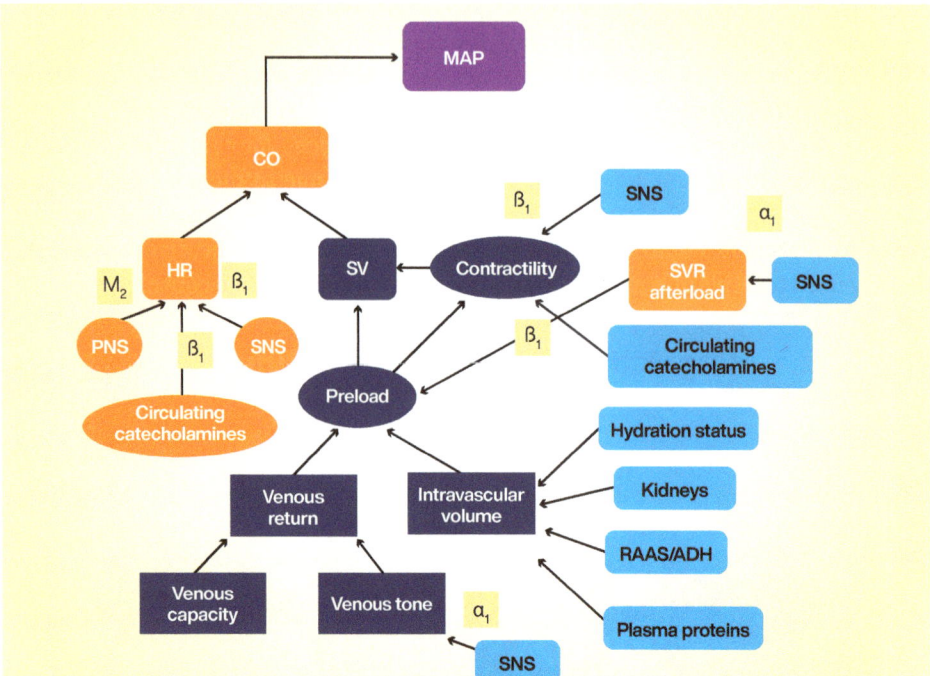

Figure 5-4: Note-Taking Decision Algorithm

In very information dense slides, it can be difficult to take notes while attempting to understand the instructor's explanation of concepts. Previewing your lecture notes or slides, listening carefully in class, avoiding taking dictation and asking your instructor questions can ensure that you develop a clear understanding of concepts. Lecture recordings can be used outside of class to supplement or correct notes that you took in class.

This slide (Figure 5-4) is presented toward the end of the class and summarizes many of the physiologic and biochemical variables regulating mean arterial pressure that were taught throughout the class. Imagine for a moment that you were presented with this exact slide in class without any prior knowledge of blood pressure regulation. How would you react? Many of the students with whom I work report feeling anxious and their "brain locking up" when shown a dense slide like this. This is a great example of what students experience when exposed to a high degree of cognitive load. Simply put, cognitive load reflects the amount of information that the brain must process in any given moment. When cognitive load and effort exceeds what your brain can handle, learning can be impaired. In fact, Janson and colleagues propose that excessive cognitive load may be a reason why note-taking may not be beneficial or can get derailed in certain circumstances.[18] In their paper, the authors identify 5 cognitive processes that are associated with successful note-taking.

1. Comprehending the lecture material
2. Identifying key points
3. Linking the material to prior knowledge
4. Paraphrasing or summarizing
5. Transforming information to a written format (writing or typing)

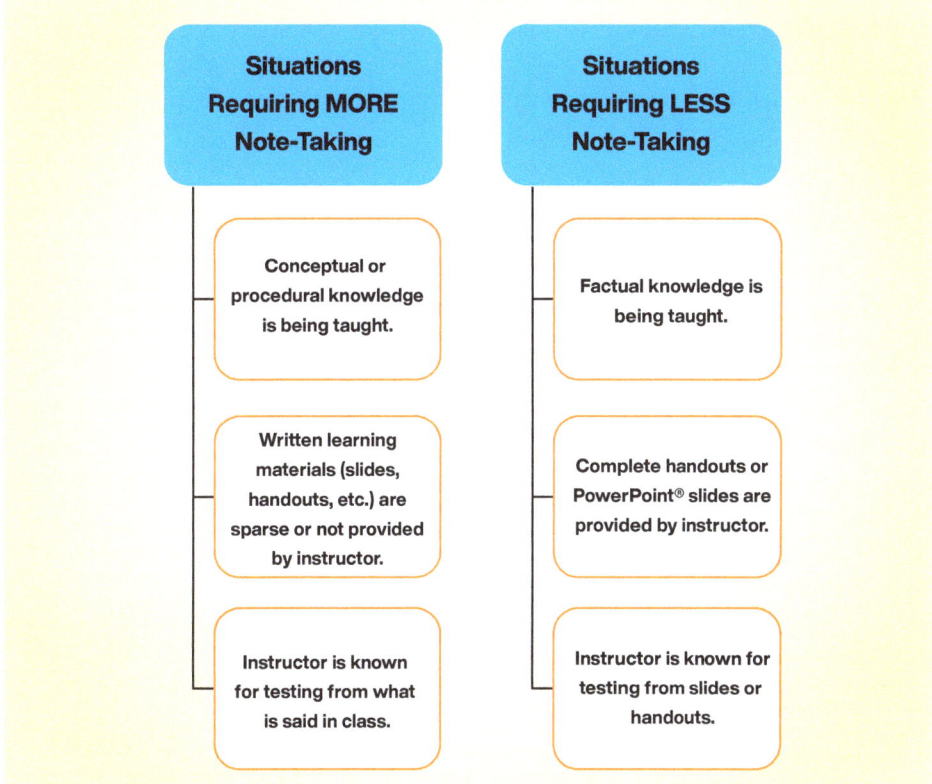

Figure 5-5: Note-Taking Decision Algorithm

Different learning situations will require different levels of note-taking. More detailed notes may be needed in courses where conceptual or procedural knowledge is stressed, learning materials like slides and handouts are not available or incomplete, or when the instructor is known for testing concepts that are described verbally in class more detailed notes may be needed. When factual knowledge is being taught, complete and detailed learning materials are provided by the instructor, and test questions typically are based on those learning materials, then fewer notes are required.

The authors argue that if one process, such as comprehension, demands an abnormal amount of mental energy, then the student is highly unlikely to engage effectively in the other four processes. If we think back to the last slide example, one can easily see the merit in their theory. I have coached many students who have had this exact experience. To overcome this type of situation, I recommend several things.

The first is making sure that you are previewing the material before class. If you come across a diagram in your textbook, handout, or slides like this, definitely spend a few extra minutes breaking it down and familiarizing yourself with it. Second, if you are still overwhelmed by this diagram after previewing, I would recommend recording this part of the lecture, taking minimal notes, and simply paying attention. Your primary goal should be to develop a basic understanding of what is being taught and ask questions if you are lost or confused. After class, go back and listen to the recorded part of the lecture focusing on that slide and take more detailed notes.

Figure 5-5 identifies some of the different variables that can help you to decide how extensive your note-taking should be.

How Should I Take Notes?

I have purposely avoided making recommendations about how to take notes for several reasons. Some of the most common note-taking methods, like the Cornell Method or outline method, may not be compatible with every class, teaching and learning strategy, or technology used to deliver or record information. That is why I think students should be flexible with their note-taking and follow some general principles rather than any one methodology. While there have been a number of recent studies looking at the purpose of note-taking, evaluating student note-taking habits, and the technology used in note-taking, there are very few studies that compare the effectiveness of common note-taking methods.[17,23-25] One of the only studies I could find on this dated back to 1971 and the results were fairly inconclusive.[26] Clearly more work needs to be done in this area; therefore, I am hesitant to recommend a specific note-taking strategy. What I hope I have done is to provide you with a better understanding of why note-taking is important, make you aware of the factors that can affect note-taking, and provide examples of circumstances where you may need to adjust your note-taking approach.

Let's summarize some of the best-practices and evidence-based approaches to getting the most out of your classroom experience.

Tip 1. Come prepared! Assuming you have completed previewing material, being in class constitutes the second exposure to the new material. Previewing helps you to develop an awareness of key concepts that will be covered in class. It may also reduce the cognitive load to which you are subjected when exposed to incredibly dense and detailed learning materials. Previeiwing will help you to pay attention and to ask appropriate questions on new or confusing material. Keep in mind that the classroom is where the process of understanding and building context begins. The more prepared you are to listen and think about explanations of difficult material, the further along you will be in achieving learning goal 2. Being prepared can also help you from becoming lost if your mind wanders or you doze off!

Tip 2. Take good notes! Prior to class, take time to evaluate any learning materials that have been assigned to you. Examine learning objectives for class, and identify the type of knowledge to which you will be exposed. Consider how detailed and dense the notes are, how familiar you are with the topic, and from what materials the instructor tests. For in-class note-taking remember that less is more. Use abbreviations for complex terms (make sure you define or record what those abbreviations mean), paraphrase and summarize what the instructor is saying, and avoid taking dictation. Use different colored pens or highlighters to help you quickly identify important concepts later. Finally, remember that note-taking does not end when class ends. You should plan to reread, correct, and clean up your notes as soon as you can after class.

Tip 3. Class recordings can be a valuable learning tool only if used correctly. Technology has made capturing and disseminating classroom content increasingly easier. While at first glance this might seem to be an important resource to enhance learning, it can have unintended consequences. Many of my newer students prepare for exams by listening to lectures in hopes of learning through "osmosis". This is a very passive, inefficient way of learning and I only recommend this strategy is if the student has a long commute between home and campus or if they are suffering from incurable insomnia! The appropriate way to use lecture recordings is as a learning supplement. If you are in lecture and your mind wanders or you do not understand a concept that is being explained, mark your notes with the general time during the recording when this happens. Once you begin reviewing your notes that evening, play that segment back. For many students simply hearing the explanation again can clear up any confusion they might have or help them to capture material they have missed.

Tip 4. Actively participate in class. For many, the term "class participation" conjures up images of the type-A student who sits in the front row of the classroom in a seat directly in FRONT of the instructor. When a question is posed by the instructor, this students frantically waves a hand as if flagging down a New York City taxi in a driving rainstorm. While this is certainly one type of class participation, it may not gain you any points with your classmates. Participating in a lecture-based class is as simple as preparing for class by previewing notes, paying attention, and thinking about what the instructor is teaching. Trying to see new information in the context of prior knowledge while also answering and asking appropriate clarifying questions are also important components of stage 2, understanding and building context. Teaching strategies like problem or team-based learning require students to be active participants throughout most or all the class. While this type of teaching strategy has been shown to be very effective and is gaining popularity with instructors, many still choose to use a mixture of lecture and active learning during class. Whatever strategy is being used, make sure you are engaged in the process. Your performance during the activity can provide you with immediate feedback about the success of your learning. Even a simple "clicker" question during a lecture can provide you with immediate and valuable feedback regarding how well you remember, understand, and are able to apply a concept you just learned.

If you make the most of your classroom experience, by the time the class is over you should be familiar with major concepts and ideas and may have already started to apply them.

Key Concepts from Chapter 5

1. **Go to class! The research in this area shows that students who attend class do better academically than those who don't.**

2. **Note-taking is important because it helps you create a durable, accurate record of what was taught in class that can be used in studying outside of class. Effective note-taking that involves deep processing of material and paraphrases or summarizes main points that are being taught can help enhance encoding of information.**

3. **Whether you take handwritten notes or type them, always makes sure you do the following:**

    a. **Reduce any distractions while note-taking (this is especially important for students using electronic devices).**

    b. **Throughout the class, make active decisions about what information to record.**

    c. **Don't take dictation! Rather, paraphrase or summarize what the instructor is saying.**

d. **Familiarize yourself with your instructors teaching style.** Take the time to review learning materials (handouts, PowerPoint® slides, book chapters, articles) and learning objectives before class. The type of knowledge being taught (factual, conceptual, or procedural), its density and, the complexity of the learning materials can all impact the amount and type of notes that you take.

4. The most important part about note-taking is what you do with those notes after class and before the exam!

REFERENCES

1. Palmer S, Chu Y, Persky AM. Comparison of rewatching class recordings versus retrieval Practice as post-lecture learning strategies. *Am J Pharm Educ*. 2019;83(9):7217. doi:10.5688/ajpe7217.

2. Annis LF. Effect of preference for assigned lecture notes on student achievement. *J Educ Res*. 1981;74(3):179-182. doi:10.1080/00220671.1981.10885306.

3. Kiewra K, Benton S. The relationship between information-processing ability and notetaking. *Contemp Educ Psychol*. 1988;13:33-44.

4. Peverly ST, Brobst KE, Graham M, Shaw R. College adults are not good at self-regulation: a study on the relationship of self-regulation, note-taking, and test taking. *J Educ Psychol*. 2003;95(2):335-346. doi:10.1037/0022-0663.95.2.335.

5. Zazulia A, Goldhoff P. Faculty and medical student attitudes about preclinical classroom attendance. *Teach Learn Med*. 2014;26(4):327-334.

6. Johnston ANB, Massa H, Burne THJ. Digital lecture recording: a cautionary tale. *Nurse Educ Pract*. 2013;13(1):40-47. doi:10.1016/j.nepr.2012.07.004.

7. Persky AM, Kirwin JL, Marasco CJ, May DB, Skomo ML, Kennedy KB. Classroom attendance: factors and perceptions of students and faculty in US schools of pharmacy. *Curr Pharm Teach Learn*. 2014;6(1):1-9. doi:10.1016/j.cptl.2013.09.014.

8. Gump SE. The cost of cutting class: attendance as a predictor of success. *Coll Teach*. 2005;53(1):21-26. doi:10.3200/CTCH.53.1.21-26.

9. Credé M, Roch SG, Kieszczynka UM. Class attendance in college: a meta-analytic review of the relationship of class attendance with grades and student characteristics. *Rev Educ Res*. 2010;80(2):272-295. doi:10.3102/0034654310362998.

10. Hidayat L, Vansal S, Kim E, Sullivan M, Salbu R. Pharmacy student absenteeism and academic performance. *Am J Pharm Educ*. 2012;76(1):8. doi:10.5688/ajpe7618.

11. Ta A, Neumiller JJ, Kim AP, Remsberg CM, Gothard MD. The effect of pharmacy students' attendance on examination performance in two sequential active-learning pharmacotherapy courses. *Am J Pharm Educ*. 2020;84(9):ajpe7749. doi:10.5688/ajpe7749.

12. Schnee D, Ward T, Philips E, et al. Effect of live attendance and video capture viewing on student examination performance. *Am J Pharm Educ*. 2019;83(6):6897. doi:10.5688/ajpe6897.

13. Westrick SC, Helms KL, McDonough SK, Breland ML. Factors influencing pharmacy students' attendance decisions in large lectures. *Am J Pharm Educ*. 2009;73(5):83. doi:10.5688/aj730583.

14. Fjortoft N. Students' motivations for class attendance. *Am J Pharm Educ*. 2005;69(1):15. doi:10.5688/aj690115.

15. Morehead K, Dunlosky J, Rawson KA, Blasiman R, Hollis RB. Note-taking habits of 21st century college students: implications for student learning, memory, and achievement. *Mem Hove Engl.* 2019;27(6):807-819. doi:10.1080/09658211.2019.1569694.

16. Kiewra KA. Providing the instructor's notes: an effective addition to student notetaking. *Educ Psychol.* 1985;20(1):33-39. doi:10.1207/s15326985ep2001_5.

17. Kiewra KA. A review of note-taking: the encoding-storage paradigm and beyond. *Educ Psychol Rev.* 1989;1(2):147-172. doi:10.1007/BF01326640.

18. Jansen RS, Lakens D, IJsselsteijn WA. An integrative review of the cognitive costs and benefits of note-taking. *Educ Res Rev.* 2017;22:223-233.

    doi:10.1016/j.edurev.2017.10.001.

19. Di Vesta FJ, Gray GS. Listening and note-taking. *J Educ Psychol.* 1972;63(1):8-14. doi:10.1037/h0032243.

20. Mueller PA, Oppenheimer DM. The pen is mightier than the keyboard: advantages of longhand over laptop note-taking. *Psychol Sci.* 2014;25(6):1159-1168. doi:10.1177/0956797614524581.

21. Fiorella L, Mayer RE. Spontaneous spatial strategy use in learning from scientific text. *Contemp Educ Psychol.* 2017;49:66-79. doi:10.1016/j.cedpsych.2017.01.002.

22. Anderson LW, Krathwohl D. *A Taxonomy for Learning, Teaching, and Assessing: A Revision of Bloom's Taxonomy of Educational Objectives.* Boston, MA: Allyn & Bacon. Boston, MA; 2001.

23. Liles J, Vuk J, Tariq S. Study Habits of Medical Students: An Analysis of which Study Habits Most Contribute to Success in the Preclinical Years. *MedEdPublish.* 2018;7(1). doi:10.15694/mep.2018.0000061.1.

24. Luo L, Kiewra KA, Flanigan AE, Peteranetz MS. Laptop versus longhand note-taking: effects on lecture notes and achievement. *Instr Sci.* 2018;46(6):947-971. doi:10.1007/s11251-018-9458-0.

25. Stacy EM, Cain J. Note-taking and Handouts in The Digital Age. *Am J Pharm Educ.* 2015;79(7):107. doi:10.5688/ajpe797107.

26. Palmatier R. Comparison of four note-taking procedures. *J Read.* 1971;14(4):235-240.

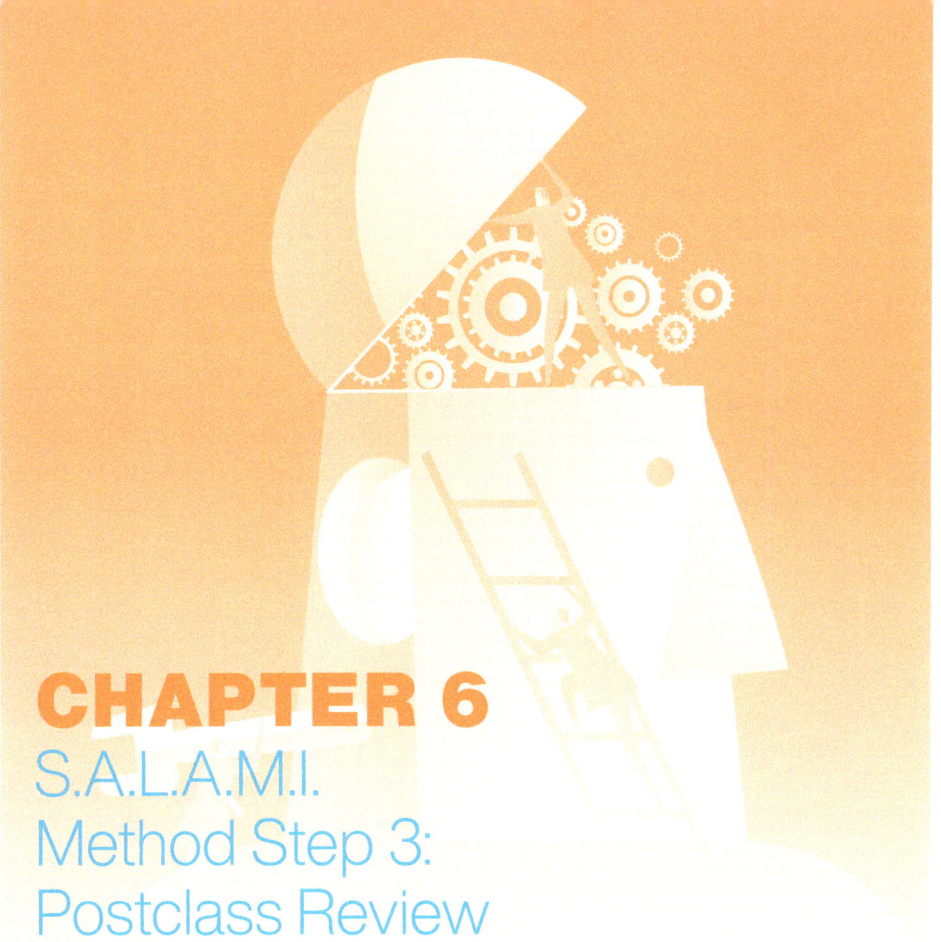

CHAPTER 6
S.A.L.A.M.I. Method Step 3: Postclass Review

Case Study
M.L. is a first-year student struggling in the pharmaceutics course. During our first coaching session, the student says that when studying, remembering anything learned in class or how to solve the example problems assigned as in-class work is a struggle. Additionally, when sitting down to study, M.L. feels lost and unsure of where to begin. As we talk, I discover that there is typically a 3 to 5–day delay before the student begins studying concepts and practicing problems that were introduced in class. M.L. wants to know what can be done to improve learning and course performance.

CASE STUDY ANALYSIS

Step 3 of the S.A.L.A.M.I. method, postclass review, is extremely important for bridging learning goal 2 (understanding and building context) and learning goal 3 (memory formation and strengthening). M.L.'s primary issue is not interfacing with the course material until several days after class and by then most of what was learned in class had been forgotten. Once M.L. starts studying, considerable time must be spent redeveloping an understanding of the material before beginning the process of encoding and consolidation. Does this sound familiar? To help address the challenge, I spent some time teaching M.L. how to engage effectively in postclass review. The analogy I like to use to explain postclass review involves bread making. Preparing for class (step 1) is analogous to collecting the ingredients necessary for bread making. In-class engagement (step 2) is analogous to mixing the dry ingredients and activated yeast together, and postclass review (step 3) is comparable to letting the dough rise before baking (step 4: preexam preparation) using a technique that I call "postviewing."

Like previewing, postviewing should not take more than 10-20 minutes. Your goal is to continue to promote memory formation through encoding and consolidation by mentally processing the material and reflecting on the recent learning experience (class). I will refer to the process used during step 3 as postviewing. This process has 5 steps.

1. *Without the aid of notes* or class materials, summarize or list the main concepts you learned in class.
2. Correct your written notes by clarifying what you have written and ensuring that it makes sense.
3. Identify tables, figures, diagrams, readings, etc. from learning materials that might require extra time to consolidate and apply.
4. List topics that you struggled to *remember and understand* from class.
5. Identify resources available to practice application of concepts.

Let's take a moment to discuss each of these steps in more depth.

Step 1. Without Notes or Other Learning Materials, Summarize or List the Main Concepts Learned in Class

Attempting to summarize or list concepts you learned in class can help you to begin the process of consolidation as well as identification of concepts that you are having difficulty remembering or understanding. During this step of the S.A.L.A.M.I. method, recalling detailed information is not the goal, rather remembering broader concepts, how they fit together, and gauging your level of understanding is. In order to complete this postviewing step, you can apply two learning strategies that are commonly used as active learning exercises in class, focused listing and the minute paper strategy. To use focused listing, simply make a list of all the concepts or facts that you remember from class. If the amount of material you learned in class is significant, it may help to generate multiple lists. For example, if you were learning about antihypertensive agents and your instructor covered, thiazide diuretics, calcium channel blockers, and ACE inhibitors, you could do focused listing on each of those three topics. Using the minute paper strategy at this stage of learning is more challenging but still reasonable. With the minute paper exercise, you set a timer for one minute and write a paragraph that describes what you learned in class. Once again if multiple topics were covered you may need to generate multiple minute papers. Keep in mind that you are most likely not going to be terribly successful at either of these activities right after class as you are still in the very early stages of encoding and consolidating information into long-term memory. The important thing to remember is that it is important to make the attempt. Even unsuccessful retrieval of information has been shown to be beneficial to the learning process compared to no retrieval practice.[1,2]

Step 2. Correct Notes by Clarifying What You Have Written, Ensuring It Makes Sense

Remember in the last chapter that note-taking does not end when you leave class! The better shape your notes are in before you study, the more useful they will be later. After class you should take a few minutes to reread your notes and make any corrections to ensure they are readable and error free. You should not recopy them. If you find there are errors or sections of notes that you don't understand, you can use class recordings to make the corrections. Simply find the section of the recording that corresponds to the notes that you took and relisten to that part. Don't fall into the trap of repeatedly listening to your lecture recordings! This learning strategy is extremely passive and does not effectively promote memory formation when compared to evidence-based learning strategies like active recall. Fortunately, many note-taking apps have a feature that will help you to avoid this by recording what the instructor is saying as you write or type your notes. All you have to do is click on the notes that you want to correct, and the app will play back what the instructor was saying at the time you took the notes. A final component of step 2 is to attempt to summarize major concepts that were taught in class, paraphrasing longer passages of notes that you might have taken.

Step 3. Identify Tables, Figures, Diagrams, Readings, etc. from Learning Materials Requiring Extra Time to Consolidate and Apply

As you are correcting your notes, make sure that you mark sections that might require extra time to learn or study. This is especially important if the instructor indicates they are important. With limited amount of time to study, focusing on items that are difficult, detailed, or deemed important by the instructor can help you use your time most effectively.

Step 4. List Topics You Struggled to Remember and Understand from Class

Step 4 is closely related to step 3 but is based on your actual class experience. After a brief review of your notes, you should begin identifying concepts that are confusing or difficult to remember by marking specific sections of handouts or slides or making a list. Identifying difficult concepts will allow you the opportunity to seek timely help from your course instructors. Eliminating knowledge gaps in a timely fashion will help to promote understanding of concepts you will learn in the future. If knowledge gaps exist, understanding more complex and closely related material that you will learn will be more difficult. By getting timely help from your instructors, you can quickly eliminate these gaps, which will make future learning easier.

Step 5. Identify and Use Resources Available to Practice Application of Concepts

Timely application practice is a powerful way to improve understanding, contextual awareness, and consolidation. It is also necessary to achieve learning goal 4, utilization. Remember from Chapter 2 that the term "utilization" is being used in the broad sense to encompass all of the higher levels of learning, creating, evaluating, analyzing, and applying. When preparing for any kind of assessment involving utilization, I believe it is important to follow these guidelines.

First, when practicing application, try to simulate exam conditions. We can gain valuable insight into how to prepare effectively for any exam that involves utilization of concepts by looking at how professional athletes and musicians prepare for sporting events and performances. Each of these groups of professionals use scrimmages or dress rehearsals to simulate the actual conditions under which they will be performing to ensure they are fully prepared. I recommend taking the same approach with any practice problems your instructor assigns.

The second recommendation is to attempt to complete practice problems under timed conditions and without the aid of learning materials or assistance from other classmates. Remember you will not have these resources available during the exam. If you can't do the problems without those resources during practice, there is little chance you will be able to do it on an exam. My students commonly work on problem sets with other students. When working on a problem in a group, every member should work independently. A set amount of time should be given for everyone to complete the problem, and once that time has expired, then the group can discuss the solution. If done correctly, valuable peer feedback and help can be gained especially if someone is struggling. While this can be an effective way to learn to work through difficult problems, setting aside time to practice solving problems and applying concepts independently is important. Evaluating your performance during these "dress rehearsals" can provide valuable feedback on your state of readiness and what you need to do to fix it.

If an instructor assigns you practice problems to complete before an examination, do not wait until the last minute to do them. Many students with whom I work make this mistake, and if they run into problems, they may not have time to get help or relearn material. My advice to the student is that it is never too early to start practicing application of concepts you are learning. Hopefully, your instructors believe this principle as well and start this process in class, providing you with problem sets or practice questions that you can work on outside of class.

What if your instructor does not give you practice problems as part of the class? In this case, you have several options. The first would be to check your textbook and online sources to find practice problems. Make sure to check that these questions cover the major concepts covered in class. When in doubt, ask your instructor to evaluate the questions. If your instructor is unwilling to do this, then vetting questions through classmates can give you some idea that you are on track. Your second option could be to inquire about using old exams given in the course. If your instructor passes exams back and allows students to keep them, then this option might be viable. I do offer a word of caution; **before you choose to use these exams, make sure you check with the course instructor to ensure that the use of old exams is permissible.** In some cases, copies of old exams might have been acquired using less than honest methods and without the knowledge or consent of your instructor. Your third option is to create your own application questions. Writing exam questions, especially those that require application of concepts takes time and is not easy. Despite this, the effort involved can help you develop a deeper understanding of the material and provide opportunities to practice application, especially if they are lacking from your instructor. Taking advantage of the knowledge and different perspectives of study group members can help to make this process easier. Drawbacks to this option include the time it takes to write the application questions, especially if you are working alone, and the applicability and correctness of questions that study partners might write.

Postview Guide Sheet

Class: _____ Date: _____

Instructions: Following the class and on the same day, work through the 5 steps listed below. This process should take no more than 10-15 minutes.

1. Without the aid of notes or other learning materials, take 1 minute to write a paragraph summarizing the main concepts you learned in class.

2. Review your 1 minute paper, and identify major topics that you struggled to remember from class.

3. List topics that you struggled to understand during class.

4. Identify tables, figures, diagrams, readings, etc. from learning materials that might require extra time to consolidate and apply.

5. List resources that are available to help practice application.

Key Concepts from Chapter 6

1. Postviewing is a useful strategy for transitioning from S.A.L.A.M.I. step 3 to step 4. At the end of each class you should take a few minutes to

   a. write a paragraph summarizing the main concepts you learned in class.

   b. correct your written notes by clarifying what you have written and ensuring that it makes sense.

   c. identify tables, figures, diagrams, readings etc. from learning materials that might require extra time to consolidate and apply.

   d. list topics that you struggled to remember and understand from class.

   e. identify resources available to practice application of concepts.

2. Timely application practice is a powerful way to improve understanding, contextual awareness, and consolidation. If an instructor assigns you practice problems to complete before an examination, do not wait until the last minute to do them.

3. When practicing problems in preparation for an exam, you should attempt to simulate exam conditions. Give yourself a set amount of time to complete the problems and do not use any learning materials to help you solve the problems.

REFERENCES

1. Richland LE, Kornell N, Kao LS. The pretesting effect: do unsuccessful retrieval attempts enhance learning? *J Exp Psychol Appl*. 2009;15(3):243-257. doi:10.1037/a0016496.
2. Grimaldi PJ, Karpicke JD. When and why do retrieval attempts enhance subsequent encoding? *Mem Cognit*. 2012;40(4):505-513. doi:10.3758/s13421-011-0174-0.

CHAPTER 7
S.A.L.A.M.I. Method Step 4: Preexam Preparation Part 1, Keys to Effective Studying

Case Study

P.T. is a second-year pharmacy student who scheduled an appointment with me in the middle of the semester because of some recent academic difficulties. The student is taking a heavy academic load including an 8-credit, integrated pharmacology, pathophysiology, and therapeutics course. P.T. has recently been elected vice president of the Student National Pharmaceutical Association (SNPhA) and is working 20 hours a week as an intern. The student admits to being completely overwhelmed and being behind with course work. P.T. feels very unproductive while studying. Finding study sessions difficult to initiate, the student is usually distracted by the cell phone after finally sitting down to study. P.T. also admits to staying up late to study and deciding what to study each day based on upcoming exams.

CASE STUDY ANALYSIS

The primary goal for step 4 of the S.A.L.A.M.I. method is building a durable working knowledge base that can be used to successfully complete pharmacy school, pass the NAPLEX and, most importantly, to provide better care for your patients. I have found that students who are the most productive in step 4 have the following characteristics:

1. **They have a focused and engaged mindset.**
2. **They take the time to develop a daily study plan using S.M.A.R.T. (specific, measurable, attainable, relevant, and time bound) goals.**
3. **They interleave studying related subject areas.**
4. **They space their study instead of blocking or cramming.**
5. **They devote a significant amount of study time to the use of evidence-based learning strategies like active recall, elaboration, or dual coding.**
6. **They use the data generated from their active recall practice to gauge the effectiveness of their study and to plan future study sessions.**
7. **They practice application of concepts.**

Unfortunately, P.T. has not yet adopted many of these approaches or developed these skills. In fact, the student's approach to learning is a great example of some of the most common ones reported as being used by struggling students. These include reacting to upcoming exams rather than being proactive with study, not planning out study sessions, and doing a lot of studying at night.[1-5] If you are using any of these approaches, then you know how easy it can be to fall behind with your learning and get caught up in a reactive study pattern. Once that happens, the cycle is difficult to break.

How did P.T. get into this situation? Certainly, a large course load and extracurricular activities have contributed to the situation; however, there are other issues at work. Take a moment and think about how you typically start a study session. Do you dive right in like P.T., or do you take some time to formulate a plan? Do you have a set of criteria that allows you to effectively choose what to study? Do you study for whatever exam is coming next or do you have a more strategic approach? Do you have a method for determining the time you are going to allocate studying a topic and know when you are ready to move on to another topic? Do you use an evidence-based approach to choosing the method that you are going to use to learn new concepts when you study? The answers to these questions can have a significant impact on your learning, and, in this chapter, we are going to explore them in more detail as I teach you a common method of goal-setting combined with two powerful evidence-based strategies, spacing and interleaving.

Spacing

One of the most critical decisions that any student will make about learning is how frequently they should study course related material. A lot of research has been done attempting to determine an optimal answer to this question. Studies to date have clearly shown that learning and retention is greatly enhanced when students spread out or distribute their study of content material. This is referred to as spacing.[6,7] A very powerful way of using spacing in your study is to combine it with retrieval practice. This combined approach is often referred to as "distributed practice" or "distributed active recall." This approach can easily be used to improve your academic performance; yet, very few students are aware of this approach, and fewer yet put it into practice.

Despite being relatively simple to understand and implement, most students do not space out their learning well. Instead they use a massed approach to studying. Using this approach, students attempt to master a large amount of information in a short period of time. Unfortunately, blocked and massed practice has been shown to be less beneficial than distributed practice especially when the focus is on long-term retention of information.[8]

One common form of massed studying is cramming. Students who engage in massed studying right before an exam, or "cramming," are not leaving themselves enough time to strongly encode information into long-term memory. I refer to this approach as the "binge and purge" method of studying for obvious reasons. While studying very close to an exam might allow you to remember a significant amount of information for a short period of time and do well on the exam, it is likely that you will end up forgetting it very quickly.[9] This can be a problem later when you are on your Advanced Pharmacy Practice Experiences (APPEs) and need to remember what you learned to take care of patients!

Blocked studying is another form of massed studying. An example of this is studying a single subject for a long period of time one day, and then waiting for four or five days to study this material again. During that four- to five-day period between study sessions, the process of forgetting begins to erode much of the learning from the first study session. Many of my students who block their study report not remembering much in between study sessions and having to start from scratch during each new study session. Figure 7-1 is a hypothetical illustration that shows the impact on knowledge retention using this type of study pattern. The bar on the left shows the amount of information retained during a single, four-hour study session. By day four, represented by the bar on the right, a significant amount of forgetting has occurred. During this second four-hour study session the student must spend a considerable amount of time "re-learning" what was studied on day one and, as a result, has less time to initiate learning of new concepts. Students who use this strategy can find, as an exam nears, they have not made much progress on their learning despite spending a lot of time studying.

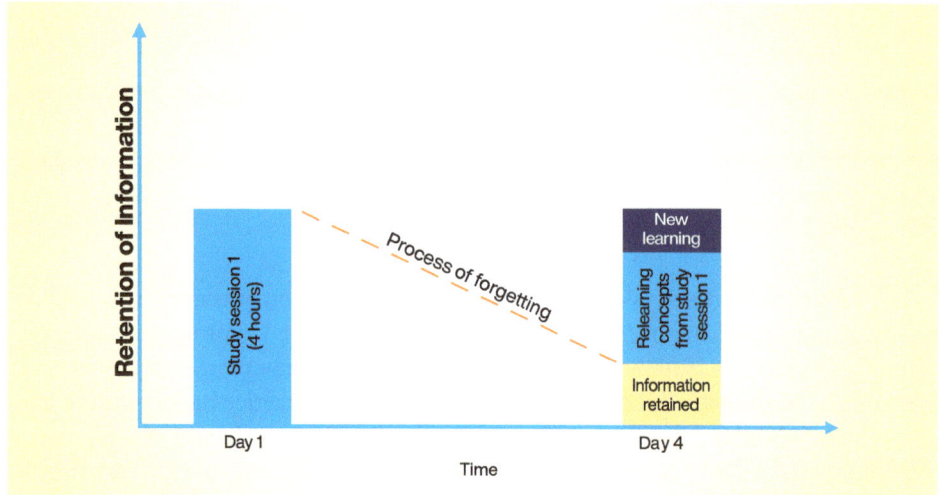

Figure 7-1: Process of Forgetting During Blocking of Study

A hypothetical diagram illustrating what happens when students block their study. When they choose to study one subject for a long period of time and then wait for a long period of time to restudy, much of the initially retained information is lost. This loss of information is sometimes referred to as the "process of forgetting."

Figure 7-2 is a hypothetical example of how spacing can be applied to your studying to enhance the effectiveness of active recall and to arrest the process of forgetting. One of the first things you notice on the graph is instead of two, four-hour study sessions separated by three days there are shorter, daily sessions that occur over the same four-day period. The total amount of study time represented in the Figure 7-1 (eight hours) is identical to the total study time represented in Figure 7-2. This is the key to spacing or distributed learning. You spend a similar amount of time studying as you would with massed or blocked study, but that time is spread out to maximize learning. You can see how the amount of knowledge retained grows as the bars progress from left to right. The most likely reasons for this are that less forgetting occurs and that the act of retrieving information from memory seems to encode information more strongly.

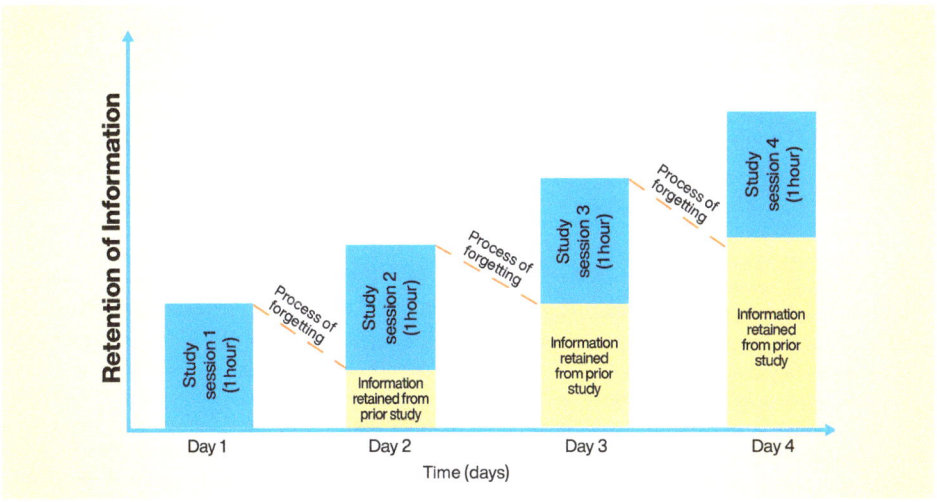

Figure 7-2: Process of Forgetting During Spacing of Study
When students space their study of a topic over regular intervals (daily) the amount of forgetting between each study session is reduced and gains in learning increase despite spending the same amount of time studying throughout the week. In addition, the amount of forgetting that occurs in between regularly spaced study sessions can help to enhance learning, especially when active recall strategies are being used.

Many successful students I have surveyed seem to use a combination of both mass practice and spacing. During the weeks leading up to an examination, they use spacing to develop a strong knowledge foundation and then switch to a mass practice mode several days before the exam. When they make this switch, they significantly increase the amount of time and attention they give to the material on the upcoming exam. It is not clear to me nor have I encountered any studies that suggest that this combination of study techniques is better or worse than spaced practice alone. I think that the secret to making this combination work is to make sure that you do not stop studying your other subjects during the mass practice phase. In the days leading up to a major exam or assessment, falling behind in your other courses is very easy. If this happens, catching up may be difficult or impossible.

Interleaving

Practicing active recall with multiple topics or subjects during a single study session is an evidence-based learning strategy called "interleaving," which can further boost long-term retention of information.[10,11] Interleaving appears to be maximally effective if subject materials are closely related and has broad applicability to many types of learners and subject areas.[12,13] The learning power of interleaving is based on making mental connections between related concepts when studying for different courses. For example, interleaving your study of pharmacology, medicinal chemistry, and therapeutics together would be particularly effective, especially if you are studying the same drugs in each of these courses at the same time. If you were learning about calcium channel blockers in all three of these courses and studied and interleaved each course during a study session that night, you would be able to connect how the chemical structure of that drug influenced its binding to specific ion channels (medicinal chemistry), how blocking those channels can lower cardiac output and vascular resistance (pharmacology), and how these drugs can be used with cardiovascular diseases like hypertension. This in turn can help to encode this information more strongly into long-term memory. Conversely, interleaving study of pharmacy management and pharmacokinetics courses would not be as effective as these topics bear little similarity to one another.

Coming Up with a Plan

Effective study session goals can be generated quickly and effectively with a little bit of practice, especially if you use the S.M.A.R.T goal format.[14] S.M.A.R.T. stands for specific, measurable, attainable, relevant, and time bound (Figure 7-3). This acronym has been used for decades in situations in which goals need to be set, achieved, and measured. It can also be a powerful tool to help making your study sessions more effective.

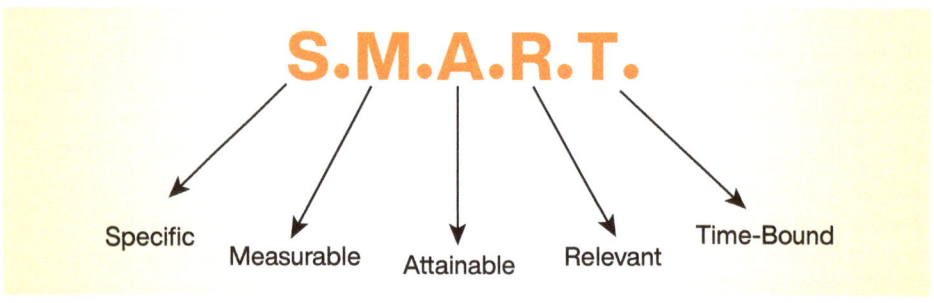

Figure 7-3: S.M.A.R.T. Goals

The acronym S.M.A.R.T. has been widely used to describe the characteristics that increase the utility of goals. Daily goal setting is an important component to any daily academic plan, and students who use the S.M.A.R.T. goal format are more likely to be more productive in their daily learning.

SPECIFIC (S)

Study session goals that are specific (S) will help you to stay on task and focus on what you need to accomplish. Study session goals should be quantitative or measurable and qualitative or descriptive when needed. Examples of quantitative goals include reviewing 10 pages of biochemistry notes, completing questions 1-5 in a pharmaceutics problem set, or reading and taking notes on 2 sections of a chapter in your physiology textbook. Goals with a qualitative component to them are more descriptive. Examples include setting a goal of completing questions 1-5 in a problem set and only using your notes or text to help you with 2 out of the 5 questions or learning 70% of the material on 10 pages of biochemistry notes.

Avoid developing vague goals like, "I want to study biochemistry, pharmaceutics, and physiology tonight." These types of goals are not very useful. Without a specific endpoint, determining when they have been accomplished is difficult.

When you are creating a study plan, make use of interleaving and spacing. When helping my students develop a daily study plan, I ask them to identify the two to three most difficult courses they are taking and make sure that they create daily S.M.A.R.T. goals around them. This helps to promote regular spaced study of these courses. If these two to three courses are related, which they often will be, you can take advantage of the interleaving effect. This can encourage thinking about how materials in different subjects are related and, in turn, help to promote understanding and retention. Consider the following example and how it applies to what we just learned.

Goals for Study Session. Example 1:
1. Study pharmacology of hypertension drugs time:
    three hours.

versus

Goals for Study Session. Example 2:
1. Pharmacology of beta blockers and ACE inhibitors
    Review: note pages 14-24
    Time allotted: 50 minutes
2. Break: 10 minutes
3. Treatment of hypertension, first line agents
    Review: note pages 52-68
    Time allotted: 50 minutes
4. Break: 10 minutes
5. Pharmacy practice management
    Read: pages 24-36 and Chapter 10 in textbook
    Time allotted: 50 minutes

Based on what we learned about S.M.A.R.T. goals, which of the two sets of goals would you chose? I hope it would be the second. The first example has several problems. First, the goal itself is very general. There is no indicator of what types of drugs are going to be studied. Secondly, only one subject is being studied in a three-hour period. This is a perfect example of blocking the study of a subject. Example 2 is a much better set of goals for studying. Each of the goals is very specific, and multiple subjects are being learned over the three-hour period, with two of them being closely related and interleaved. The interleaving occurs when the pharmacology of calcium channel blockers and ACE inhibitors is studied for one hour followed immediately by the therapeutic application of these drugs in hypertension. Understanding the mechanism of action of a drug can help you to understand why and how it is used in a patient and why it can cause specific side effects. Understanding the inhibitory of effects of ACE inhibitors on bradykinin breakdown can help you understand better why some patients develop cough and make it more likely to remember that information. Putting both subjects in context with one another can help facilitate a deeper understanding of each individual subject and promote better retention of information.

MEASURABLE (M)

Being able to measure (M) or determine the attainment of your goals for the study session is very important. Quantitative study goals, like the examples above, are straight forward to measure. You either did problems 1-5 or you did not. You were either able to do three out of five problems without external assistance, or you were not. When we are talking about measuring learning goals, however, it is not enough to just check a box after we have studied a subject on our list. We need to be able to gauge the success of our learning. A simple way to accomplish this is through the use of active recall methods. Active recall is an important evidence-based learning strategy, and we are going to look at several ways you can incorporate this into your study in Chapter 8. Whatever strategies you do use, you must examine the results of your effort and use that to inform future studying.

ATTAINABLE (A)

Developing study goals that are not attainable (A) is one of the most common and critical mistakes that students make using the S.M.A.R.T approach to goal setting. Your study goals should be realistic and achievable in the time allotted. If you expect to read and digest sixty pages of your microbiology text or encode and consolidate into long-term memory twenty pages of pharmacotherapeutics notes in a one-hour period, you are setting yourself up for failure. On the other hand, if you leave yourself too much time to complete a certain study task, you eliminate a sense of immediacy that is important to learning and may make it difficult to keep up with the rapid pace of most classes.

One way to ensure that your goals are attainable is to triage those goals based on their level of importance, deadlines, and your aversion to completing them. When I was little, I didn't like to eat vegetables at dinner. Most of the time I would eat everything I liked first and by the time I got to my vegetables they were cold. Unfortunately, I was not allowed to leave the dinner table until I had finished them. My parents urged me to eat my vegetables first while they were hot as they tasted much better. I urge you to keep this advice in mind when you study. Studying for courses that you may not like or that you may not be doing well in first, allows you to use your fresh reserve of energy, focus, and concentration while leaving favorite or easy classes for later that require less of these mental resources to study. Either way, determining whether a goal is achievable or not in the allotted time is a metacognitive skill that takes time to develop. It requires consistent practice, self-evaluation, and a clear knowledge of one's ability to learn. Fortunately, this skill is one that you can develop rapidly and will significantly improve the efficiency of your study sessions.

RELEVANT (R)

Another important consideration is the relevancy (R) of your study session goals. There are three questions that are important to ask when considering what to study.

1. What subjects are you going to study?
2. What component of those subjects are you going to study or work on?
3. What specific learning materials are you going to use?

There are many variables that you might have to consider when deciding what to study. Your top two to three most difficult courses should be on your list regularly. Upcoming assessments may also have an impact on your choice of what to study and for how long. When deciding what subjects to study, remember the principles of spacing and interleaving that we have already discussed. Use the results of your active recall attempts to assess what you know is important. A strong self-awareness of what you know is an important part of metacognition development and can help you be more efficient in your studying. Many students with whom I work tend to restudy material that they have already mastered and avoid material with which they are struggling. The reason they do this is because they rely on their feelings rather than real data to tell them how well they know a concept. Overstudying information that you already know can give you a false sense of accomplishment and knowing, preventing you from working with material with which you might be struggling or on which you are behind. Data about how well you have mastered a concept can be gained from monitoring the results of active recall attempts. In Chapter 8, I teach you an active recall method called the Boxing Technique. One of the strengths of this technique is that it generates real-time data about the degree of mastery you have developed with material in your lectures. You can use this data to make decisions about your future study, which can save you a lot of time.

Finally, studying the appropriate material is critical to maximize your learning. I have worked with several students over the years who made it a habit to ignore most handouts, slides, and other learning materials created by course instructors in favor of learning from someone on YouTube. While it is true that hearing someone explain a difficult concept in a different way can be helpful, you must be sure that that person has the qualifications to explain the material and that their descriptions are correct. Just keep in mind that most instructors I know spend many hours carefully crafting learning materials for their students. In addition, these materials are designed to focus on the knowledge, attitudes, and skills that the instructors want their students to acquire. In this case, why would you study anything else?

TIME BOUND (T)

Each of your study goals should have a self-imposed time limit associated with it. Assigning time limits to tasks creates a sense of immediacy, promotes focus on task, allows for interleaving and distributed practice, and prevents resorting to mass practice techniques that are not effective.

The following are a few S.M.A.R.T. goals that could comprise a single three-hour study session:

1. **Retrieval practice on information for pages 1-5 of biochemistry notes that you studied the previous night. Identify and review concepts that you are having difficulty retrieving. (20 minutes)**
2. **Study pages 15-25 of biochemistry notes and practice retrieval of knowledge on basic concepts about transcription and translation. (30 minutes)**
3. **10-minute break**
4. **Complete problem set questions 1-7 in pharmaceutics. (50 minutes)**
5. **10-minute break**
6. **Write draft reflection on recent health fair experience. (30 minutes)**
7. **Use drug flash cards to study the first 20 of the top 200 drugs. (20 minutes)**

Engagement and Focus

Effective studying and learning are hard work, and the amount of focus and commitment that you bring to your study session can have a significant impact on your learning. Being engaged and focused on task is critical to get the most out of your study session. Student athletes or musicians often have an intimate understanding of what I am talking about. Their experience practicing for a sport or rehearsing a piece of music gives them a clear point of reference. If you have no experience with music or sports, ask a student athlete or musician what it is like to participate in a practice or rehearsal. Good coaches and conductors are very efficient. During practice or rehearsal no time is wasted and there is little tolerance for goofing around. Everything that is done is purposeful and linked to a specific goal. In addition, they often hold scrimmages or dress rehearsals to provide an opportunity to practice skills under controlled, "real-life" situations. If you are having a difficult time conceptualizing the focus and commitment necessary during a productive study session, think about what level is required during an examination.

None of us possess an endless supply of focus, and when we are tired and stressed the supply that we do have is even more limited. During study there are several tricks that you can use to increase the amount of focus that you have with you. These include

1. **Dividing individual study sessions into smaller chunks of time.**
2. **Scheduling multiple short breaks**
3. **Reward yourself for achieving goals.**
4. **Using multiple retrieval practice strategies when studying.**
5. **Eliminating distractors.**
6. **Ensuring that you get enough sleep.**

There should be a sense of immediacy in your studying and having time bound tasks is a great way to develop this immediacy. If your mind is wandering or you are relaxed or having fun, you are probably not as engaged as you should be and not getting good return on your time investment. Your job is to achieve the goals that you have set in the time allotted.

Even with a high level of focus and motivation, students can easily become distracted. Smart phones, computers, social medial, texting, etc. are all competing for the limited "attention bandwidth" that we possess. These distractors can easily overwhelm your working memory. Working memory is the part of memory that stores facts and information for short periods of time while it is being processed or manipulated, and it has a limited storage capacity.[15] If you are distracted during your studying by TV, music, text messages, social media, or the Internet, you can easily lose focus and occupy one of these slots with unnecessary sensory information. When we allow these types of distractors into our study sessions, we are handicapping ourselves by allowing them to interfere with our learning.

The bottom line is that you should do everything possible to limit distractions while studying and to stay as focused as possible. If you are not mentally fatigued at the end of your study session, you are probably not as engaged as you should be. If you are having trouble staying engaged and focused during your study sessions, some of the following suggestions may help:

1. Identify an accountability partner.
2. Set aside a specific time each day specifically for studying and additional, but separate, times to engage in activities that would normally be distracting (e.g., social media).
3. Get enough sleep at night and maintain a normal sleep schedule.
4. Exercise.
5. Utilize effective time management strategies.
6. Schedule breaks and limit lengths of study sessions.
7. Reward yourself for achieving your study goals. Positive reinforcement is a critical part of maintaining motivation.
8. Allow your body and mind to adapt to the intensity and duration of study sessions. Over time it will get easier.

PROCRASTINATION

Procrastination is a type of avoidance behavior that despite its negative consequences can derail even the most determined, purposeful student.[16] At one point or another, most of us have been affected by this strange malady, which when contracted, can cause us to spend hours seeking out pleasurable, immediate rewards like watching cat videos on YouTube or scrubbing the bathroom floor with a toothbrush instead of studying.[17] Unfortunately, as enjoyable as cat YouTube videos might be, they aren't going to help you prepare for you next Pharmacokinetics exam! It is clear from the research in this area that procrastination can have a significantly negative impact on your academic performance.[18,19] Academic procrastination can be associated with anxiety and is generally characterized by a desire to delay study until the last minute, forcing the student into a situation where cramming is necessary to prepare for an upcoming exam.[20,21]

There are a number of great resources available to help even the most dedicated procrastinator. One in particular that I really like is a review article published in *Frontiers In Psychology* by Dr. Frode Svarrtdal and colleagues.[22] In their article, they outline nine different recommendations for beating procrastination. Many of these recommendations are directly related to knowledge and skills that you are learning from this book! I have taken the liberty of condensing their recommendations down to six. Let's look at some of these and see how they relate to what you have learned so far.

1. Take the time to learn about and develop metacognitive skills, specifically in the areas of planning (macro and micro time management, choosing a study space, developing S.M.A.R.T. goals), monitoring (using the results of active recall practice, data generated from exam wrappers [Chapter 9] and preexam checklists), and regulating (changing how you study based on data generated from monitoring strategies and your knowledge of evidence-based learning strategies) your learning.

2. The third, fifth and sixth recommendations have to do with learning about and using evidence-based study skills to replace inefficient study techniques. If you have made it this far in the book you are well on your way to achieving this goal.

3. Identify and eliminate distraction and temptations. Study distractors include anything that prevents engagement in focused, purposeful study. While distractors can be student and circumstance specific, I have found that the two most common types involve technology and other human beings. Technology based distractors include portable technology such as cell phones, laptops, or tablets. Human distractors can include well-meaning family members, significant others, friends, roommates, or fellow students. Once distractors are identified, measures should be taken to eliminate them from the study environment. Your list of distractors should be visibly present during each study session and reviewed before any work begins.

4. Look for and recognize even small success and victories and reward yourself for them!

5. If you are engaged in a study group, make sure that it is efficient and effective. If group members insist on using passive, ineffective learning strategies, encourage them to use evidence-based ones or find a new group!

6. Study with individuals who are performing at a level which you would like to achieve. You will be surprised at how you can rise to the occasion.

You must remember that while how much you study is important, what you do while you study is even more important. As you plan your study sessions, use high-impact learning strategies like retrieval practice. Avoid low-impact strategies like recopying notes, listening to recorded lectures, reading, and highlighting.

OVERLEARNING

Another trap that students fall into is overlearning. Overlearning occurs when students continue to study information even after they have developed mastery.[23,24] While under certain circumstances overlearning can have benefits, especially when skills are being learned that are best done without much conscious thought, there are some practical downsides when it comes to studying.[25] Overlearning can easily happen with introductory material presented at the beginning of a block of instruction. As students return to review introductory material daily, they develop feelings of comfort and familiarity that reinforces their desire to continue to study that material. This in turn leads to the illusion of productivity and promotes, supports, or reinforces avoidance of harder material that might be more difficult to master. The result is an inadequate understanding of more difficult concepts and those that are taught closer to the exam.

Assessing your performance on retrieval practice and problem-solving activities during studying can help you avoid overlearning. If you are successful in these activities, without using notes, textbooks, or other learning materials, then it is time to focus on other material. Revisiting mastered information before the exam is appropriate, but the time you should spend reviewing it should be regulated. As a rule of thumb, the better your mastery of material, the less frequently you should be studying it.

Key Concepts from Chapter 7

1. Interleaving and spacing are two evidence-based strategies that you can use not only to plan out your study but also to help enhance the encoding of information into long-term memory.

2. S.M.A.R.T. goals are a great way to structure and develop a daily study plan. These types of goals are specific, measurable, attainable, relevant, and time-bound.

3. To improve your engagement and focus during study sessions try dividing individual study sessions into smaller chunks of time, scheduling multiple short breaks, rewarding yourself for achieving goals, using multiple retrieval practice strategies when studying, eliminating distractors, and ensuring that you get enough sleep.

4. To avoid academic procrastination, invest time in learning about and using metacognitive and evidence-based learning strategies, eliminate as many distractors as possible, recognize even the small victories, make sure your study group is productive, and study with those whose academic performance you would like to match.

REFERENCES

1. Kornell N, Bjork RA. The promise and perils of self-regulated study. *Psychon Bull Rev*. 2007;14(2):219-224. doi:10.3758/BF03194055.
2. Yan VX, Thai KP, Bjork RA. Habits and beliefs that guide self-regulated learning: do they vary with mindset? *J Appl Res Mem Cogn*. 2014;3(3):140-152. doi:10.1016/j.jarmac.2014.04.003.
3. Hartwig MK, Dunlosky J. Study strategies of college students: are self-testing and scheduling related to achievement? *Psychon Bull Rev*. 2012;19(1):126-134. doi:10.3758/s13423-011-0181-y.
4. Geller J, Toftness AR, Armstrong PI, et al. Study strategies and beliefs about learning as a function of academic achievement and achievement goals. *Memory*. 2018;26(5):683-690. doi:10.1080/09658211.2017.1397175.
5. Persky AM, Hudson SL. A snapshot of student study strategies across a professional pharmacy curriculum: are students using evidence-based practice? *Curr Pharm Teach Learn*. 2016;8(2):141-147. doi:10.1016/j.cptl.2015.12.010.

6. Cepeda NJ, Pashler H, Vul E, Wixted JT, Rohrer D. Distributed practice in verbal recall tasks: a review and quantitative synthesis. *Psychol Bull*. 2006;132(3):354-380. doi:10.1037/0033-2909.132.3.354.

7. Carpenter SK, Cepeda NJ, Rohrer D, Kang SHK, Pashler H. Using spacing to enhance diverse forms of learning: review of recent research and implications for instruction. *Educ Psychol Rev*. 2012;24(3):369-378. doi:10.1007/s10648-012-9205-z.

8. Dunlosky J, Rawson KA, Marsh EJ, Nathan MJ, Willingham DT. Improving students' learning with effective learning techniques: promising directions from cognitive and educational psychology. *Psychol Sci Public Interest* 2013;14(1):4-58.

9. Hartwig MK, Dunlosky J. Study strategies of college students: are self-testing and scheduling related to achievement? *Psychon Bull Rev*. 2012;19(1):126-134. doi:10.3758/s13423-011-0181-y.

10. Birnbaum MS, Kornell N, Bjork EL, Bjork RA. Why interleaving enhances inductive learning: the roles of discrimination and retrieval. *Mem Cognit*. 2013;41(3):392-402. doi:10.3758/s13421-012-0272-7.

11. Dobler IM, Bäuml KHT. Retrieval-induced forgetting: dynamic effects between retrieval and restudy trials when practice is mixed. *Mem Cognit*. 2013;41(4):547-557. doi:10.3758/s13421-012-0282-5.

12. Hausman H, Kornell N. Mixing topics while studying does not enhance learning. *J Appl Res Mem Cogn*. 2014;3(3):153-160. doi:10.1016/j.jarmac.2014.03.003.

13. Yan VX, Sana F. The robustness of the interleaving benefit. *J Appl Res Mem Cogn*. 2021;10(4):589-602. doi:10.1016/j.jarmac.2021.05.002.

14. Doran GT. There's a S.M.A.R.T. way to write management's goals and objectives. *Manage Rev*. 1981;70(11):35-36.

15. Miller EK, Buschman TJ. Working memory capacity: limits on the bandwidth of cognition. *Daedalus*. 2015;144(1):112-122. doi:10.1162/DAED_a_00320.

16. Klingsieck KB. Procrastination: when good things don't come to those who wait. *Eur Psychol*. 2013;18(1):24-34. doi:10.1027/1016-9040/a000138.

17. Dryden W. *Overcoming Procrastination*. London, England: Sheldon Press; 2000.

18. Rozental A, Carlbring P. Understanding and treating procrastination: a review of a common self-regulatory failure. *Psychology*. 2014;05(13):1488-1502. doi:10.4236/psych.2014.513160.

19. Steel P. The nature of procrastination: a meta-analytic and theoretical review of quintessential self-regulatory failure. *Psychol Bull*. 2007;133(1):65-94. doi:10.1037/0033-2909.133.1.65.

20. Steel P, Klingsieck KB. Academic procrastination: psychological antecedents revisited. *Aust Psychol*. 2016;51(1):36-46. doi:10.1111/ap.12173.

21. Limone P, Sinatra M, Ceglie F, Monacis L. Examining procrastination among university students through the lens of the self-regulated learning model. *Behav Sci*. 2020;10(12):184. doi:10.3390/bs10120184.

22. Svartdal F, Dahl TI, Gamst-Klaussen T, Koppenborg M, Klingsieck KB. How study environments foster academic procrastination: overview and recommendations. *Front Psychol*. 2020;11:540910. doi:10.3389/fpsyg.2020.540910.

23. Rohrer D, Taylor K. The effects of overlearning and distributed practise on the retention of mathematics knowledge. *Appl Cogn Psychol*. 2006;20(9):1209-1224. doi:10.1002/acp.1266.

24. Dougherty KM, Johnston JM. Overlearning, fluency, and automaticity. *Behav Anal*. 1996;19(2):289-292. doi:10.1007/BF03393171.

25. Driskell JE, Willis RP, Copper C. Effect of overlearning on retention. *J Appl Psychol*. 1992;77(5):615-622. doi:10.1037/0021-9010.77.5.615.

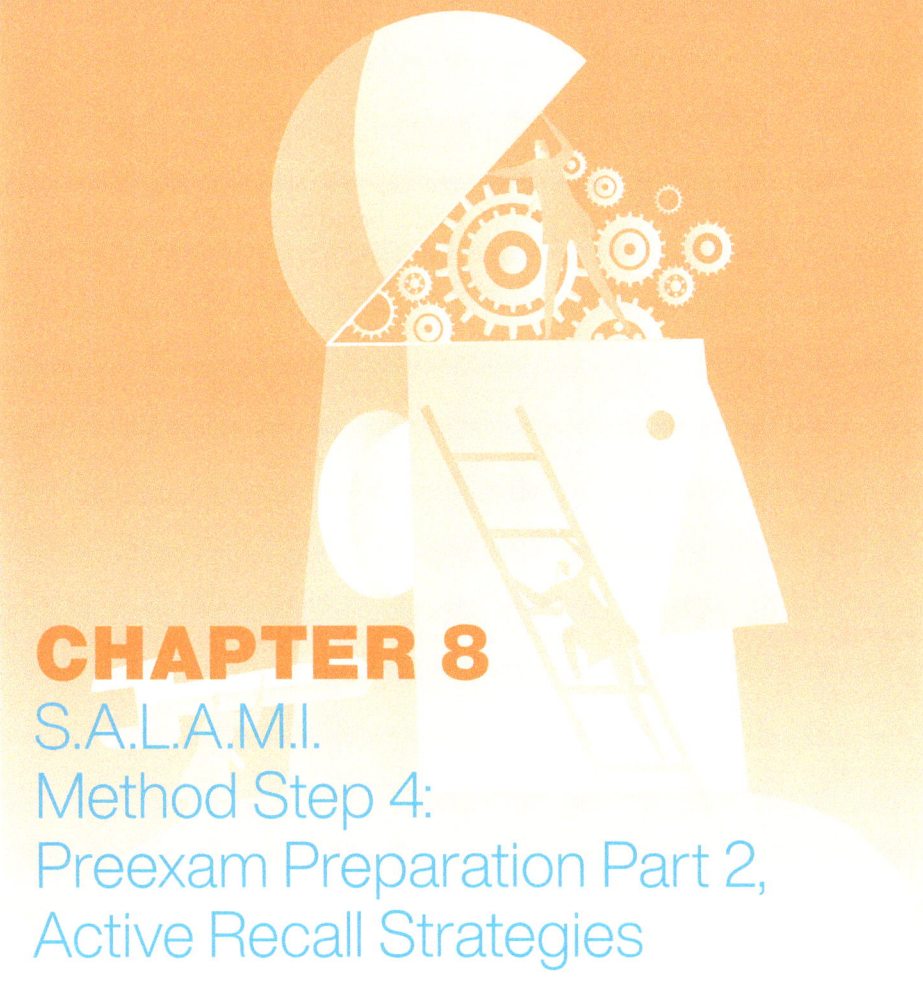

CHAPTER 8
S.A.L.A.M.I. Method Step 4: Preexam Preparation Part 2, Active Recall Strategies

Case Study

C.W. is a second-year pharmacy student who has consistently performed at a C-level since starting the program. During our initial academic coaching session, the student admits to being extremely frustrated with exam performance. "Dr. Culhane, I study at least 20 to 30 hours a week, and every time I get an exam grade back, I am disappointed. Going into the test, I always think that I am going to do better than my final grade reflects. Most of the multiple-choice questions I miss are because I narrow my answer to two selections and usually pick the wrong one. I am also terrible when 'select all that apply' is one of the answer choices. I usually get most of the answer correct but am always missing a part of the answer that causes me to get the whole question wrong!"

CASE STUDY ANALYSIS

C.W.'s complaint is one that I have heard from hundreds of students over the course of my career and is representative of two major issues that I see with learners: the inability to accurately predict their exam grades based on their perceived learning from studying and the inability to accurately recall and use information on an exam. Both issues can have a big impact on academic performance. However, there are solutions!

C.W.'s inability to predict an accurate exam grade is associated with a phenomenon that has been widely studied by cognitive psychologists called "judgments of learning" (JOLs). Judgments of learning are simply defined as our ability to gauge how much we know about something.[1] Poor JOLs are seen when students like C.W. think they know more than what their exam grades demonstrate and are commonly referred to as "the illusion of knowing or knowledge,"[2] "the illusion of competence," or "the familiarity trap." Whatever you call it, being able to accurately judge your knowledge in a particular area, especially before testing, is critical for productive studying.[3,4]

Poor JOLs are typically thought to be the result of deficits in students' metacognitive monitoring, which we discussed in Chapter 1. If you remember, metacognitive monitoring is the ability to gauge the effectiveness of learning during study.[5] As it turns out, most human beings, including pharmacy students, are very bad at determining what they know or don't know.[6] To make matters more complicated, our inability to accurately judge our level of learning appears to be influenced by a number of factors including poor academic performance, a desired grade on an exam, or perceived beliefs about how much we know about a specific topic.[7,8] I have found that most student's illusion of knowledge is a result of relying on their feelings of learning rather than actual data they generate while they are studying. Fortunately, using active recall strategies when studying seem to help alleviate poor JOLs.[9] I am going to teach you an active recall method called "the boxing and unboxing technique" that will help you to easily track the success of your learning by generating actual data to better gauge how prepared you are for an upcoming assessment.

There are two other clues that tell me a lot about the cause of C.W.'s frustrations. Provided C.W. is accurate about the time spent studying each week, a major issue challenge that we need to work on is something I refer to as the "illusion of productivity." The illusion of productivity is very common in students, especially when they begin academic coaching with me. At the center of this trap are several key characteristics. The first is the belief that regardless of what you do while studying, the more time you spend, the more you learn and the better you will perform on an exam. The second is overestimating the productivity of your study sessions-

study sessions, which reinforce the feeling that you have accomplished a lot just because you spent a long time studying. Lastly is a complete lack of knowledge of evidence-based learning strategies.

When explaining how the illusion of productivity and its characteristics work to students, I use the following analogy :

Imagine your job is to go outside and dig a six-foot-deep hole. To do this, you decide to use a spoon. You spend the next ten hours digging with the spoon. Over those ten hours you will have done a lot of work will be tired and dirty and may feel extremely productive. How much real progress do you think you have made? Now imagine if I took your spoon, gave you a shovel, and taught you how to use it. How would that change what you are able to accomplish and how you feel about it?

The second clue is C.W.'s inability to recall facts and information in enough detail to answer multiple choice questions, especially the "select all that apply" variety. Typically, when I work with students like C.W., I quickly uncover that they are using very passive and unproductive methods to study like reviewing their notes, recopying notes, listening to lectures, and condensing notes and memorizing them. They may also lack focus and goal orientation. If you see some of yourself in C.W., then using the information presented in this chapter can help your learning significantly.

Reviewing Your Notes

As I mentioned before, one of the passive, ineffective study strategies that many students use is reviewing or rereading their notes. This is a method of study that I do not recommend as a primary mode of studying and ideally should constitute only a small part of your overall study plan. If you are going to take time out of your study session to review notes, make sure that you avoid the common mistake of reading your notes in the same way that they might read a magazine article, blog, or web page. This type of passive, surface reading will only promote a passing familiarity with the material that can easily be confused with mastery. If you have to review or read your notes, it is better to use more active strategies to engage with the material, like this paper they contend that successful students tend to interact with written material using numerous active strategies.[10] These strategies can be adapted to help students interface more effectively with their class notes or other learning materials. When reviewing your notes try to

1. Anticipate and write test questions that can be used for future active recall.

2. Attempt to paraphrase and summarize what is written in lecture handouts.

When doing this, be careful that you are using appropriate language and that you are factually accurate.

3. Remember that context is critical. Don't make the mistake of viewing your notes or other classroom material as a collection of unrelated facts. Think about the facts contained in these informational sources as pieces of a large puzzle. Each piece has its own unique size, shape, and colors; however, on its own, it has little meaning or usefulness. Only when we actively put it into place with other pieces do we begin to see the bigger picture. When reviewing your notes look for connections between concepts you are studying as well as knowledge that you have gained from other classes.

4. Focus on developing an understanding of the meaning and relationship of the material you are studying rather than memorizing facts.

5. Use concept maps, diagrams, or pictures to translate written text into a graphic representation of the material.

6. Engage in active recall!!!!

Active Recall

Simply put, active recall, is one of the single most important techniques that you can use to improve your learning. This evidence-based strategy goes by several names including "self-testing" and "retrieval practice" and involves repeatedly accessing or retrieving information from memory. The positive memory effects of active recall have been known for over a century and have several benefits.[11] First, research has shown that active recall strengthens memory and long-term retention of material.[12-14] It also provides you with important information about the status of your own learning that can be used to modify study efforts in the future. The more time a student devotes to this process, the easier for the brain to "locate" and utilize a fact or piece of information. I often explain the importance of this component of learning to students through this analogy.

Imagine you have a treasure chest full of gold that you want to hide by burying it in the middle of a forest. You take your chest and a shovel, walk into the woods, and bury the chest. You walk out and don't revisit the site for another two weeks. How easy do you think it would be to find that buried chest? If you are able, it would probably take you some time to find the spot where it was buried. Now, if you revisited that site daily, you would become more familiar with landmarks. You might even wear a path into the forest floor, and each trip to the spot would take less and less time.

Repeatedly accessing information through retrieval practice, like going to the buried chest on a regular basis, helps to solidify information, or the path to the chest, in long-term memory. This in turn allows your brain to access the information more quickly, which is especially important on timed examinations or other types of assessments.

There are several basic components to successful retrieval practice. Retrieval practice should constitute a significant part of your study time. As a high-impact learning strategy, active recall is one of the most effective methods for encoding information quickly and efficiently into long-term memory and can maximize the return on your investment of time in studying.

Retrieval practice should be varied, especially if there are long periods between exams. Do not make the mistake of using the same retrieval tool or technique repeatedly. This can lead to mindless drilling of information. By varying the types of retrieval practice that you use, you can avoid memorizing information and promote consolidation. I usually recommend multiple retrieval practice strategies to my students when there is more than two weeks in between course exams.

Retrieval practice should be effortful. The more difficult it is for you to recall information, the more benefit you will receive from that practice.[15] Think about it in this way: if you go to the gym for two hours to lift weights and you only use very light ones, you are not going to see significant gains in your strength and you will have wasted a lot of time. If, however, you use heavier weights that challenge your muscles, you will see much faster and larger increases in your strength. This is a basic concept used by athletes to train their bodies for competition. Challenging your mind and body to do more difficult tasks can improve your performance in the classroom and on the field. One of the ways to make active recall more challenging and effective is to space out your retrieval attempts. Empirical studies have shown that to get the maximum benefit from this technique, enough time should pass between active recall attempts to allow you to forget some of the information. This forgetting of information introduces what is called a desirable difficulty into learning.[15] A common question I get from my students is how much time I should let pass between active recall attempts. The answer, unfortunately, is complex. Some of the research in this area suggests that one day may be optimal, and this is generally the time frame that I recommend to my students as it seems to fit well into a student's typical study pattern.[16-18] Other studies have been unable to determine an optimal spacing of time.[19,20] The important point is that the vast majority of research in this area points to spacing out your study and active recall over regular intervals is far more effective than cramming or blocking when long-term retention is the goal for which you are striving.[21]

During active recall you are going to make mistakes and fail to remember facts, concepts, and how to apply them. This is going to make you feel uncomfortable and frustrated. This is completely normal. Don't make the common mistake of avoiding active recall because of these negative emotions. Making mistakes while you learn is hugely important for learning, and making mistakes "during practice" and having a chance to correct them is much better than making them for the first time on an exam.

Done incorrectly, active recall may cause you to overestimate your learning.[22] To avoid this, you should attempt to mimic exam conditions and engage in active recall without the aid of your notes, textbook, or other learning materials. These learning materials should only be used to verify the accuracy of the information that you are recalling.

Students with whom I work often struggle to identify ways in which they can practice retrieval of information while studying. Inspiration can be found in the form of active learning strategies that your instructors may have used in your classes. In-class active learning strategies are designed to help students begin the process of encoding information through basic application and recall. While these activities are commonly used in the classroom, there is no reason why you can't use them during study sessions. As an added benefit, if you have classroom experience with these techniques, then you already understand how to use them.

The following are examples of some active learning strategies that that can be easily adapted for active recall purposes during study sessions. The key to successfully using these active learning strategies is to vary their usage. Getting fixated on one type of retrieval practice is easy, especially as you get good at it. Active recall is only effective if it is effortful and challenging, and some of the active learning strategies discussed below are easier than others. I typically recommend using easier strategies as you initially learn new concepts and increase the difficulty as you begin to develop mastery. At the end of this chapter, I introduce you to an alternate active recall strategy that incorporates several of the active learning strategies below, uses several evidence-based learning strategies, and will help you to track your learning daily so that you can make data-driven changes to how and what you study. This technique is called "the boxing and unboxing technique" and my students love it. If you choose to use this method, it can replace all of the active-learning strategies discussed below.

COVERING UP YOUR NOTES

This is one of the simplest and easiest forms of retrieval practice. It can be used in situations when you have limited time to study or are just beginning to work on mastery of material. To use this strategy simply cover up information with your hand or piece of paper and attempt to recall that information. When you are finished, uncover the notes and check your answer for depth, breadth, and accuracy. While this strategy may help with retrieval of specific facts or concepts, it will do little to help you with the deeper understanding that is required for application and use of knowledge.

FOCUSED LISTING

You might remember the technique of focused listing from Chapter 4. In that section, we used focused listing to activate prior knowledge and begin building context. This technique can also be used during your study sessions to help assess and promote retention of information. Focused listing requires you to identify, recall, and list key concepts from a lecture. This technique is particularly effective when you have just learned new material. Focused listing can also be used throughout preexam preparation; however, your lists should grow in length, complexity, and organization with each recall attempt. For example, let's say you are learning about β-antagonists in a pharmacology lecture. When you start studying this class of drugs outside of lecture you can use the focused listing technique to practice retrieval of information. Your list may initially look something like this as you begin studying this topic:

Beta antagonists
1. Examples: metoprolol, propranolol, labetalol
2. Block beta receptors that are G protein-coupled receptors (GPCRs)
3. Slow heart rate
4. Can cause exercise intolerance

As you move further along in the consolidation phase of learning, your list should grow in length and detail.

Beta antagonists
1. Examples: metoprolol, propranolol, labetalol
2. Block beta receptors that are GPCRs
3. Slow heart rate by reducing the slope of phase 4 of a pacemaker cell action potential
4. Can cause exercise intolerance
5. Uses: hypertension, antiarrhythmic, chronic management of heart failure
6. Reduces adenylyl cyclase activity and reduces cyclic adenosine monophosphate (cAMP) levels
7. Reduces cardiac contractility by reducing intracellular calcium

As you complete the consolidation phase of learning, your list should incorporate the final details, and, through organization, demonstrate an understanding of how the facts are interconnected.

Beta antagonists
1. Examples
    a. metoprolol
    b. propranolol
    c. labetalol

2. Uses
    a. hypertension
    b. antiarrhythmic
    c. chronic management of heart failure

3. Selectivity
    a. propranolol ($\beta 1$ and $\beta 2$)
    b. metoprolol ($\beta 1$)
    c. labetalol ($\alpha 1$ $\beta 1$ $\beta 2$)

4. Molecular Effects
    a. Equilibrium competitive antagonists at beta receptors
    b. Block beta receptors (GPCR)
    c. Coupled to Gs
    d. Reduces adenylyl cyclase activity and reduces cAMP levels

5. Physiologic Effects
    a. Slow heart rate by reducing the slope of phase 4 of a pacemaker cell action potential
    b. Reduces cardiac contractility by reducing intracellular calcium
    c. Reduces the rate of electrical conductance through the atrioventricular (AV) node

6. Side Effects
    a. Bradycardia
    b. Heart block
    c. Exercise intolerance

Remember that no matter how complex and detailed your lists are, they should always be generated by memory and checked for depth, breadth, and accuracy using your notes, textbook, or other learning materials.

EMPTY OUTLINE ACTIVITY

The empty outline activity is another great technique for practicing retrieval of information and assessing your knowledge level so that you can better direct future studying efforts. This technique may also be helpful for students who are having difficulty seeing the hierarchy or superstructure of a note set or book chapter. The empty outline activity typically is most effective in courses where large amounts of information are presented regularly and with an instructor who provides students with clearly structured handouts or slides following some type of outline format. The first step in the empty outline technique is to take an electronic copy of your handout or slides and begin to delete specific pieces of information so that you are left with only major topic headings. A before and after example is shown here.

Before
Types of Cardiac Cells

I. Autorhythmic (Pacemaker Cells)

A. Types
  1. Sinoatrial (SA) nodal cells
  2. AV nodal cells
  3. Cells of the ventricular conducting system

B. General characteristics of autorhythmic (pacemaker) cells
  1. Can generate spontaneous action potentials
  2. Highly dependent on Ca^{2+} for depolarization
  3. Important ion channels
      a. HCN (Na^+/Ca^{2+}) channels (phase 4)
      b. T-type Ca^{2+} channels (transient channels) (first half of phase 0)
      c. L-type Ca^{2+} channels (second half of phase 0)
      d. Voltage gated potassium channels (phases 3 and 4)

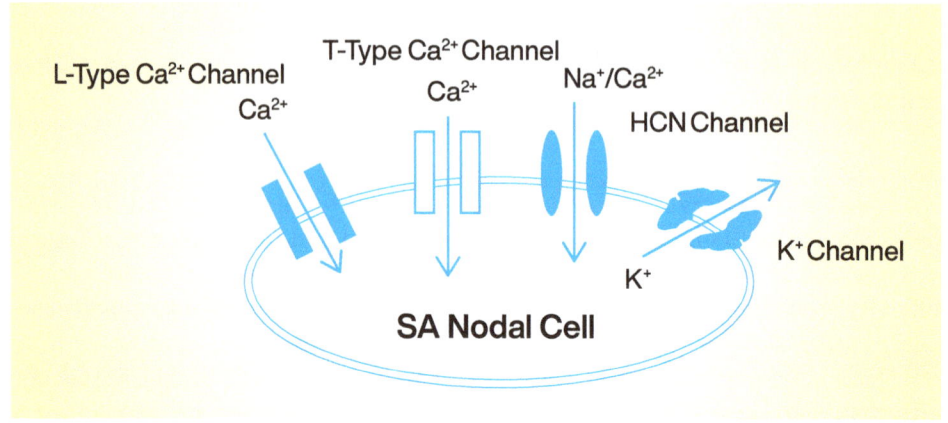

After

Types of Cardiac Cells
I. Autorhythmic (Pacemaker Cells)
    A. Types (3)
        1.
        2.
        3.
    B. General characteristics of autorhythmic (pacemaker) cells
        1.
        2.
        3. Important ion channels
            a.
            b.
            c.
            d.

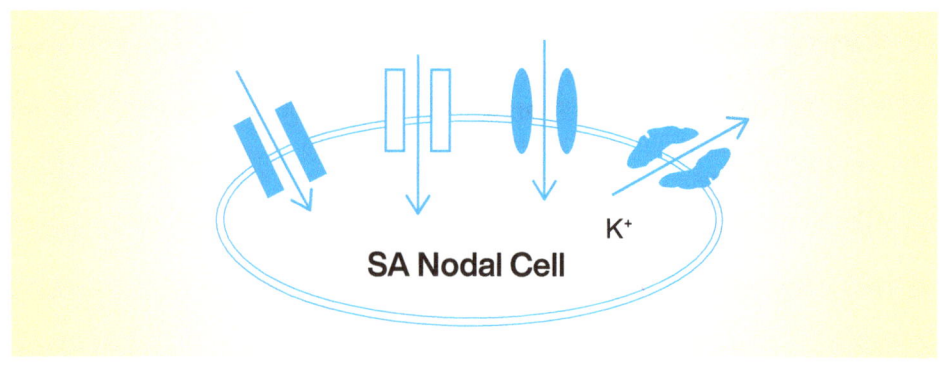

The blank outline you have generated becomes your retrieval tool. Let's imagine that learning the material on this page of notes was your goal for a study session. Once you have filled in as much information as possible, pull out your notes and self-check what you filled in. Empty spaces or incorrect information should be noted, and attention should be paid to those facts during the next study session. You should repeat this process at regularly spaced intervals until you can fill in the outline without gaps or mistakes. One of the disadvantages of the empty outline technique that my students have reported is that it can take a long time to "empty out" a set of lecture notes.

QUESTION WRITING

Writing exam questions to test your understanding and recall of information is a powerful retrieval practice strategy. It provides you with multiple opportunities to practice recall of information as well as to apply information that you have learned during the question writing process. It also can help you to get better at identifying key concepts in your classes by learning to anticipate what the exam might cover. When using the question writing strategy, make sure you have a blank sheet of paper next to you. As you read through your notes, evaluate the material to identify major concepts. Then create a question that will help you to self-test on the material later. These questions can be multiple choice, true or false, or short answer format. They can require simple recall or higher levels of thinking and processing. Writing and answering basic recall questions is most appropriate when you begin studying material. As you continue to repeatedly practice material over several days or weeks, your increased knowledge will allow you to create more complex questions that require application of concepts. These types of questions should focus on comparing concepts as well as application of material. Think about starting these questions with how, what, why, where, when, and who. One of the benefits of this technique is that the questions you develop can become part of an active recall tool that can be used again and again until you are tested and after any assessment to help reactivate prior knowledge as when you are preparing for a final exam or the North American Pharmacist Licensure Examination® (NAPLEX®).

The second way to utilize the question writing activity is to study your notes for a defined period. Close your notes and generate as many questions as possible about the material that you can think of. Attempt to answer those questions. Once completed, open your notes and check your questions and answers for **relevance and accuracy**. Below is an example of a page of notes about cardiac cell types and some examples of questions that could be generated for study.

Types of Cardiac Cells

I. Autorhythmic (Pacemaker Cells)

A. Types
   1. Sinoatrial (SA) nodal cells
   2. AV nodal cells
   3. Cells of the ventricular conducting system

B. General characteristics of autorhythmic (pacemaker) cells
   1. Can generate spontaneous action potentials
   2. Highly dependent on Ca2+ for depolarization
   3. Important ion channels
      a. HCN (Na+/Ca2+) channels (phase 4)
      b. T-type Ca2+ channels (transient channels) (first half of phase 0)
      c. L-type Ca2+ channels (second half of phase 0)
      d. Voltage gated potassium channels (phases 3 and 4)

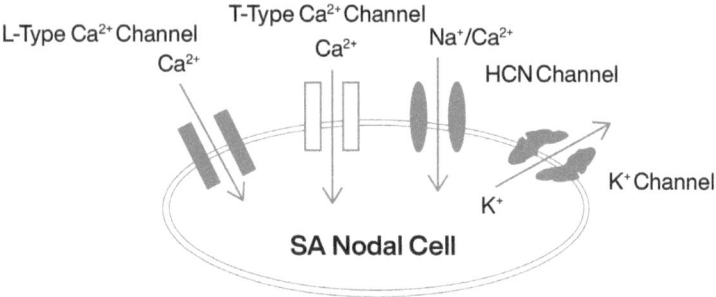

Examples of Questions

1. What are the 3 types of autorhythmic cells?
2. Describe the difference between pacemaker and nonpacemaker cells.
3. List the different ion channels autorhythmic cells use to generate action potentials.
4. Predict the impact of blocking calcium channels on the action potential generated by an autorhythmic cell.
5. Match the following ion channels with the corresponding phases of an autorhythmic cells action potential:

   Phase 0   K+ channels
   Phase 3   HCN Channels
   Phase 4   L-type calcium channel
                    T-type calcium channels

CONCEPT MAP

Concept maps can be particularly helpful in demonstrating the interrelationship between facts and ideas, as well as the organization and hierarchy within a set of notes, PowerPoint® presentation, or book chapter. Creating concept maps while studying necessitates deep thinking and processing of the material. It requires that you identify key points, determine how those points are related to one another, and create a diagram that demonstrates those relationships. Concept maps can be used in several ways during learning and using them strategically and correctly can enhance your learning.

Concept maps can be helpful if you are trying to make sense of a particularly difficult text or concept or if you are trying to untangle a confusing, disorganized, or technical handout or presentation. The goal of these concept maps is to bring order to disorder and to identify key concepts and their relationship with one another. When creating these types of maps, you will be using your notes or other learning materials. Let's consider an example of a concept map (Figure 8-1) that was created from previous example notes describing autorhythmic cells. At the center of the concept map (blue circle), we have the core concept that we are learning, autorhythmic cells. Spidering out from this circle, we have four tan boxes that represent 4 general characteristics of the autorhythmic cells that we are trying to learn: anatomical location, ion channels used, action potential characteristics, and differences from nonpacemaker cells. Finally, off these we have navy blue squares and rectangles that contain details associated with the tan squares and rectangles. There are also several colored, dotted lines that show the connection between seemingly disparate concepts. For example, there are orange, dotted lines connecting Phase 0 with the 2 ion channels that are responsible for this part of an autorhythmic cells action potential, T- and L-type calcium channels. Using a variety of geometric shapes, colors, and lines to represent concepts and their interrelationships helps create a more useful concept map.

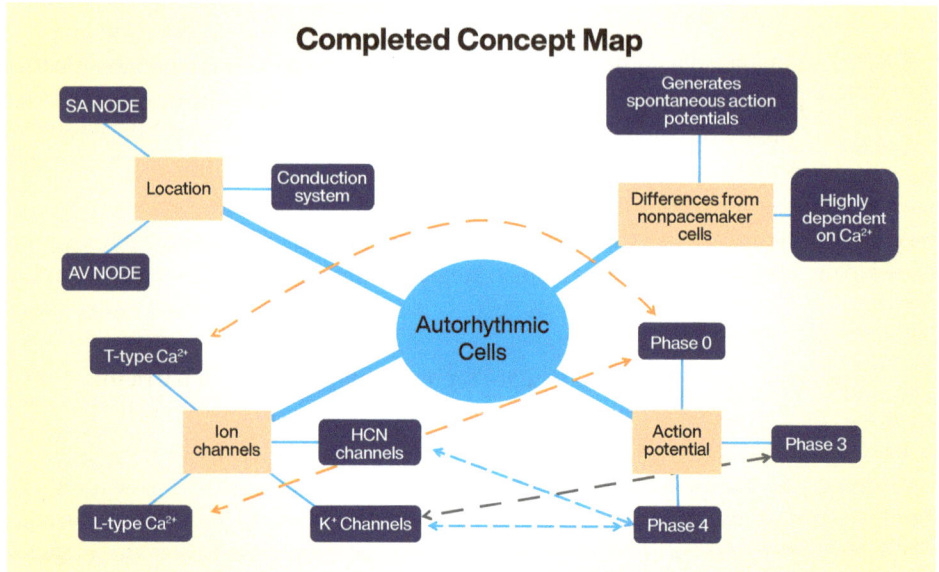

Figure 8-1: Concept Map Showing Biochemical and Electrophysiologic Characteristics of Autorhythmic Cells

This main concept map can be emptied out to use for active recall purposes. The complete concept map can be used as a self-check tool.

The second way to use a concept map is as an active recall tool. Here again, how you use the concept map is very important. Several studies have shown that the encoding effect of just creating a concept map and using your learning materials as cues, is much less effective than if you attempt to recreate the concept map entirely from memory.[23,24] This means that creating concept maps completely from memory seems to be the most effective way of using this technique to encode information into long-term memory. For many of my students, however, recreating complex concept maps from memory at first can be so hard and frustrating that they just abandon the technique all together. Remember that with active recall, hard is good and being frustrated is okay, as it indicates that learning is occurring.[15] If, however, this level of difficulty is preventing you from actively trying to recall information on your concept map, then I recommend modifying this approach in the following way and gradually work up to complete recall from memory.

Take the concept map that you initially created and eliminate some of the detail. I call this emptying out the concept map. This can be extremely easy if you initially used PowerPoint® to create your concept maps, as they can be easily manipulated to create multiple retrieval tools. If you created your concept maps by hand, you may need to redraw them. Once the retrieval concept maps are generated, you should work to fill in the missing details. Let's look at two examples of concept maps as retrieval tools. In the first example (Figure 8-2) you are only asking yourself to recall the first level of information. Do you remember what the four characteristics of an autorhythmic cell are that we covered above?

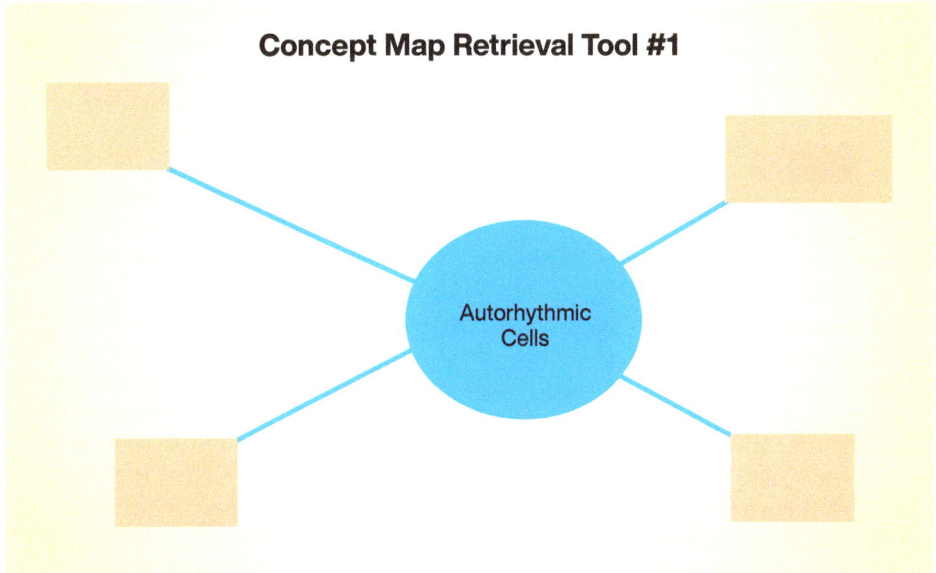

Figure 8-2: Active Recall Concept Map Showing Basic Level Biochemical and Electrophysiologic Characteristics of Autorhythmic Cells

A simple concept map can be used for initial active recall purposes. The complete concept map can be used as a self-check tool.

In the second example (Figure 8-3) you can see that the second level of detail has been added, represented by the navy blue squares and rectangles. Completing this version of the concept map will be more challenging as you need to recall additional levels of detail and information to fill in these squares and rectangles. If you want to make this even more challenging, see if you can add the arrows to the diagram.

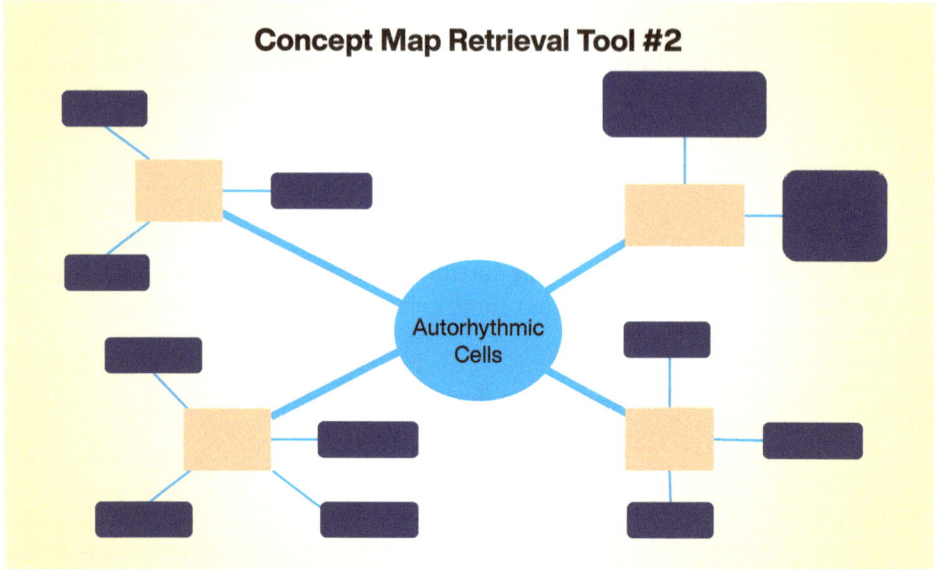

Figure 8-3: Active Recall Concept Map Showing Basic Level Biochemical and Electrophysiologic Characteristics of Autorhythmic Cells

A more complex active recall concept map requires recall of greater detail. The complete concept map can be used as a self-check tool.

Once you have finished filling in the details in any of your emptied-out concept maps, you can use your original concept map to do a self-check. This is extremely important as you should quickly correct any errors in your active recall attempt. You can also mark the concept maps to identify areas where you recalled the information erroneously or where you could not remember the information at all. This information can then be used to guide future study and to track your learning.

There are two things I want to caution you against when using concept maps for studying. The first is not to spend a lot of time creating elaborate, perfect concept maps. Those readers with an artistic flair understand what I am talking about. These are not meant to be works of art but rather tools that you can use to enhance your learning. Remember that the more time it takes for you to create a concept map, the less time you have for active recall. Another mistake I see students make with this technique is that they copy their original over multiple times, thinking that will help them to remember the concepts. This is a very passive use of concept maps and much less effective than when you use them for active recall.

MINUTE PAPER

The minute paper is an active learning technique commonly used by instructors to help students practice summarizing important concepts they learned in class. One of the key features of the minute paper is that students must recall information that they learned, determine what they think is important, and, in their own words, describe how this information is interrelated. Generating a minute paper requires *generation and elaboration*. Generation requires you to use your knowledge base to generate a paragraph describing a topic you are learning. Elaboration is a process by which you describe a concept in your own words. Minute papers or other type of writing exercise may be difficult to complete, but the challenge they provide and the effort they take to complete are well worth it.

Minute papers are very adaptable and can be used to practice retrieval from a page of notes or several slides or for complex topics. For the notes used in the empty outline example, a minute paper might look something like this:

Autorhythmic cells have the unique ability to generate spontaneous action potentials and are, therefore, responsible for pacing the heart. There are three cardiac structures that normally contain autorhythmic cells. These are the SA node, AV node, and the cells of the ventricular conducting system. Autorhythmic cells generate action potentials using several unique ion channels. These include L- and T-type calcium channels, HCN channels, and K+ channels. Each of the channels participates in 1 of 3 different phases of the action potential generated by an autorhythmic cell.

Once you have written a minute paper, you should go back to the notes to determine if there is any missing or incorrect information. Take a minute to reread the minute paper above and then review the notes in the empty outline section. What facts are missing? Does it contain incorrect or incomplete information? The process of self-assessing what you have written is as important as the writing itself. The review component of this exercise helps you to determine what information you have learned and what knowledge deficiencies exist. Unlike simple recall of facts or lists, the minute paper requires that you understand the material and can summarize the main points.

One important rule of retrieval practice is that it should be varied. It is less effective to use only one of the active learning strategies listed above. Overuse of any one active learning strategy can lead to automaticity, especially if it is used extensively for long periods of time. Automaticity occurs when you become so familiar with a retrieval practice strategy that responses to practice questions or exercises becomes automatic. This commonly happens with students who exclusively use flashcards when studying. It is one thing to be able to use your working knowledge base to answer an unfamiliar question that is written on one side of a card. It's entirely different to recognize the question as one you have read before and remember the answer that is printed on the other side. One way to avoid automaticity is to vary the type of retrieval practice you use each day. One day you might use the empty outline activity, the next the minute paper, and the focused listing after that. By changing up the type of retrieval practice you are forcing your brain to think about and recall material in different ways. This can also help you avoid mindless repetition and drilling of information that promotes short-term storage of information and rapid forgetting. Varying the types of retrieval practice, interleaving different subject material into one session, and spacing out retrieval practice are all proven strategies for increasing long-term retention of knowledge.

BOXING TECHNIQUE

The boxing technique is an active recall strategy I have developed in conjunction with my students. What makes this technique so powerful is that it is a combination of several of the active recall strategies already mentioned and it requires the use of several additional evidence-based learning strategies like elaboration, spacing, and concrete examples. One of my students who was learning to use the empty outline technique came to one of his coaching sessions reporting that emptying out his lecture was taking a lot of time. Instead of deleting text, he began to use the insert shape function on PowerPoint® to draw solid boxes on top of material on which he wanted to self-test, and the technique was born. My students and I began to refer to the technique as the "boxing technique" because of the squares and rectangles used to cover or "box up" important information on the slides. As time progressed, I added several features to the technique including an elaborative question writing component and a color-coding scheme to help monitor learning. The boxing technique seems to be very effective in classes in which a lot of factual information must be learned quickly. It has become my students' favorite technique because of its many benefits. It is easy to learn and use. It combines all the retrieval practice techniques already discussed and incorporates several evidence-based learning strategies to include active recall and elaboration. It also can help develop metacognitive monitoring by teaching the student to track learning progress using a simple color-coding system.

To implement the first step of the boxing technique in PowerPoint® or Word®, open a slide or page in your handout and take a few minutes to review the information on the screen as well as the notes that you took in class. If your notes are poor, the slides disorganized, or if you have confusion about the slide content, you may want to also listen to the corresponding part of your class recording to gain clarity. As you are doing these things, think about what your instructors emphasized. Did they take the time to provide an example of the concept about which they were talking? Did they ask you to practice using this information in class? Did they repeat the explanation of a concept several times? These are all good indicators of must-know concepts and will help you make good decisions about what information to cover up. Then use the insert shape function to cover up information on which you want to self-test in the future with colored squares or rectangles, which from this point on I will refer to as boxes, despite their lack of any three-dimensionality. The box color that I recommend that students use during this initial part of the technique is blue. The blue color indicates that no attempt has yet been made to retrieve that information from memory.

There are many ways to box out a slide. In Figure 8-4, we see examples of three different approaches on the same slide. In example 1, nine different-sized boxes are used to cover up important information in the slide. In example 2, the same slide is boxed out using only three rectangles. In example 3, one big box is used to cover up the entire slide. While there is no wrong way to box out a slide, I generally recommend using more boxes rather than just one or two. The reasons for this will become evident as we talk about the other aspects of the boxing technique.

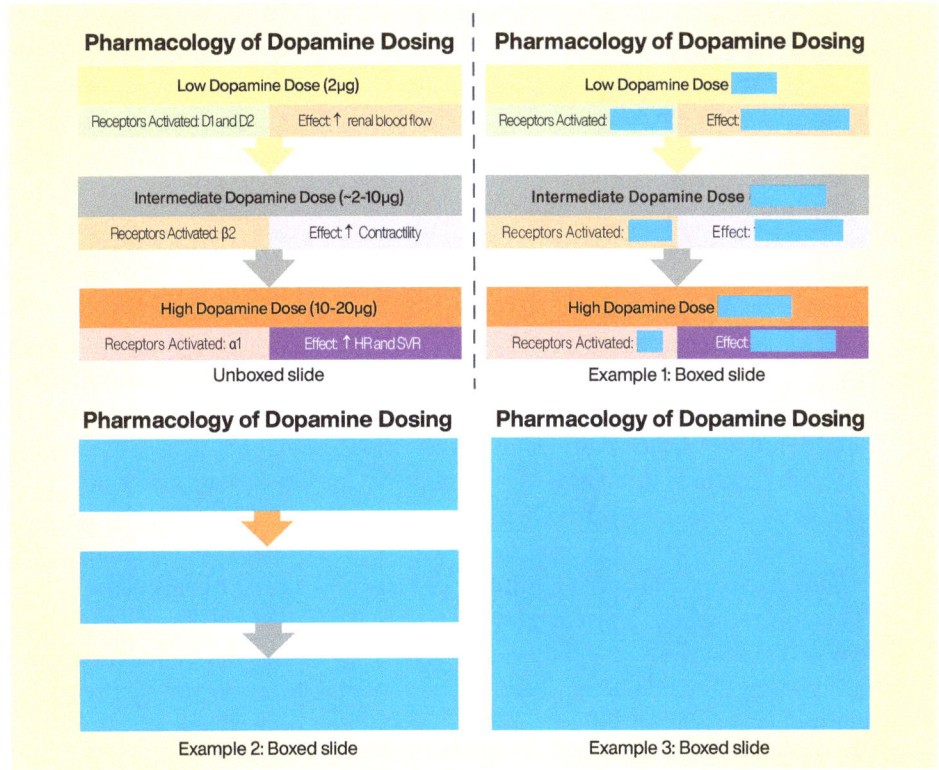

Figure 8-4: Step 1 of Boxing Technique

Use the shape drawing function in PowerPoint® or Word® to draw squares or rectangles over information which you want to practice active recall.

Once the slide is boxed out, you can begin the next step of the boxing technique, which involves adding retrieval cues to the inside of each of the boxes. This part of boxing out the lecture shares has many similarities to the exam writing active recall strategy I described earlier. Retrieval cues are questions that aid in the recall and use of the information under the box and are an extremely important part of this technique. Inserting retrieval cues is as simple as clicking on and typing text into the box.

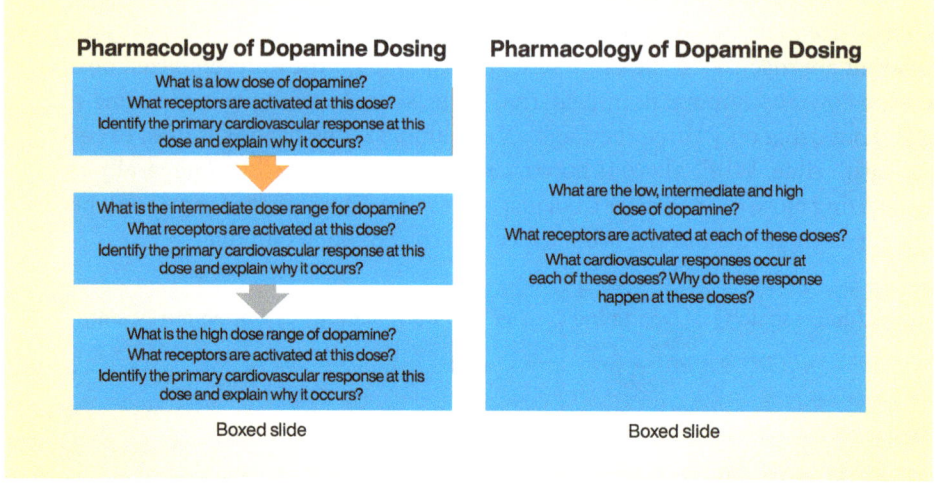

Figure 8-5: Step 2 of Boxing Technique

Retrieval cues are typed into squares or rectangles over information for which you want to practice active recall. These cues should be linked to learning objectives and ask both basic recall and application questions.

Writing good retrieval cues is the key to the effectiveness of the boxing technique and requires you to (1) have a basic understanding of the material you are boxing out, (2) make strategic decisions about what to box out, and (3) create retrieval cues that are in alignment with the learning objectives your instructor provided. The closer your retrieval cues mirror the types of questions you might see on an assessment or you might need to remember when engaged in patient care, the more effective they will be. In Figure 8-5, I have inserted retrieval cues into the boxes of examples 2 and 3. These retrieval cues are based on actual learning objectives from a class I teach in heart failure and reflect the knowledge about dopamine I emphasize to my students. Read through the retrieval cues and you will see that some require basic recall of information (i.e., dopamine dose, receptors activated, and primary cardiovascular effects). The other retrieval cue requires you to explain why each cardiovascular response occurs at a specific dose of dopamine. If your class learning objectives are focused on your ability to remember facts (identify the five side effects for drug X), then your retrieval cues in the boxes should be written in a way that supports that outcome. If the learning objectives indicate that you need to understand, apply, and evaluate the information presented, then your retrieval cues must be more sophisticated. Remember that how, why, what, where, and compare and contrast questions are the most effective and can help with deeper processing of the material.

When all your slides or note pages are boxed out and you have inserted your retrieval cues, you are ready for the last step of this technique, which we call "unboxing the lecture." To complete this step, simply start at the beginning of the slide set or handout and self-test by trying to answer the retrieval cues in each of the boxes. As you recall the information, you can speak the answers out loud or write the answer down on a piece of paper. Both are forms of the evidence-based learning strategy called "elaboration." Next, click on the blue box and move it to the side so that you can check your responses for depth, breadth, and accuracy. If you can't answer any of the retrieval cues in the box, change the color of the box from blue to red. This will help you remember during a subsequent retrieval practice session that you were unable to remember any of the information under that box. If you successfully retrieve some of the information or only partially answer a question in the box, change the color of the box from blue to yellow. In this case, changing the color of the text under the box that you had difficulty retrieving to red as an important marker for the next time may be more helpful. If you can successfully retrieve all the information under the box, change the box color to light green. Increase the shading to a darker green every time you go back and successfully retrieve the information. Remember that successfully retrieving information once or twice does not mean it is fully encoded in your long-term memory. I have found with most of my students that multiple successful retrieval attempts are necessary for this to happen. Sometimes a green box may have to be turned back to yellow or red if you can't successfully recall the information.

The color-coding system is a critical part of this technique as it will help develop your metacognitive monitoring and regulation. The different colors will allow you to quickly identify areas of strength and weakness. This in turn will allow you to be more strategic with your studying, especially as you get closer to your assessment. You can easily identify and allocate more time to areas of weakness and avoid overlearning areas where your learning is stronger.

While there is no right or wrong way to box out the information on a slide, some approaches will provide you with better information than others. Let's take a moment to revisit the two boxed-out examples of the dopamine pharmacology slide (Figures 8-4 and 8-5). Pretend that you practiced active recall on both slides and, in both cases, you were unable to successfully remember the following information: (1) the receptors activated at a low dose of dopamine, (2) the high-dose range for dopamine, and (3) the receptors activated at those high doses and the cardiovascular responses associated with a high dopamine dose. As a result, you changed the box colors to indicate what you knew and did not. Now let's examine Figure 8-6. Which of the boxed-out slides provides you with more information about your level of learning? The color-coding information given by the slide on the left is much more useful as it allows you to quickly target areas that are problematic. The large yellow box on the right just indicates that you only know some of that information but does not identify that information.

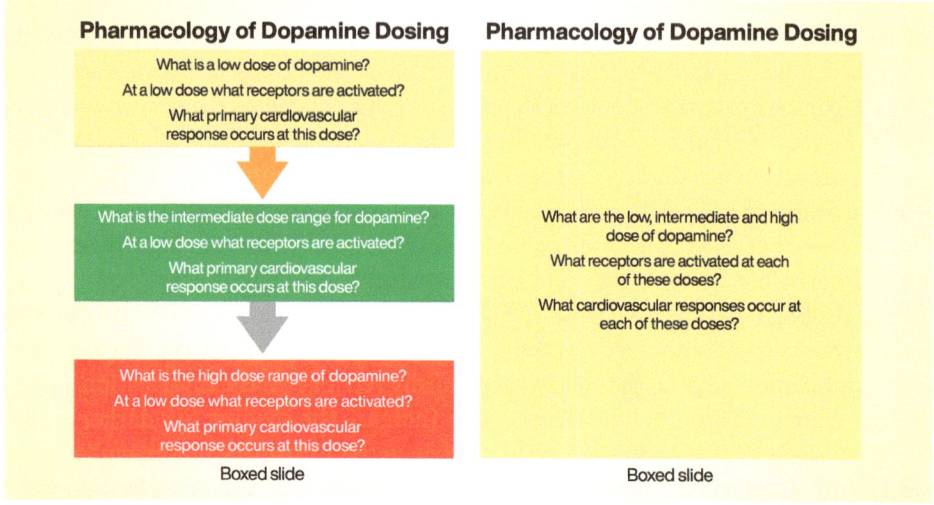

Figure 8-6: Step 3 of Boxing Technique

Unbox the lecture by attempting to answer the retrieval cues in the box, uncovering the information underneath to self-check your answer. Change the color of the box to indicate how successful you were with your active recall. Red boxes indicate you were not able to recall any information, yellow boxes indicate successful recall of some of the information, and green boxes indicate success recall of all of the information. Different shades of green can also be used to indicate how many times the information has been successfully recalled.

PowerPoint® has a very useful function that can help you to monitor your learning progress on a slide set while using the boxing technique. It is called "the slide sorter view." At the bottom right-hand corner of your PowerPoint® screen, you will see multiple icons that allow you to switch between different views to include normal, reading view, slide show, and slide sorter. When you click on the slide sorter view and zoom the screen out you should be able to see all or most of the slides in the presentation. This "birds eye view" can help you to locate quickly slides with which you are struggling so that you can be strategic with your studying. This becomes very important as you get closer to an exam or assessment. The color coding of the boxes is a critical metacognitive component of this technique as it helps you monitor in real time what you know and what you don't. As you move closer to an assessment for which you are preparing, you can be more strategic with what you are self-testing, focusing on remaining reds and yellows.

One of the most important things that I stress with my students as I teach them the boxing technique is that after your first retrieval practice attempt, you are going to have a lot of red and yellow boxes. That's OK! As you continue to practice retrieval, the colors of your boxes are going to shift from red to yellow and green. Remember that one successful retrieval attempt does not mean the information is fully consolidated in your long-term memory. This is especially important if you attempt to unbox your learning materials immediately after study. Waiting for some time to pass after you have boxed out your learning materials before you attempt active recall is best. Many of my students, when they first start using the boxing/unboxing method, will immediately begin active recall after they finish boxing out a slide set. As such, they tend to do very well and, as a result, develop a false sense of knowing. I always recommend allowing a day to pass after boxing out a lecture before you begin unboxing it with active recall. This allows enough time for a little forgetting to occur, which will make active recall challenging but not enough to make it impossible. Effective memory encoding and consolidation requires successful retrieval of information multiple times over the time-period in which you are studying for an exam (days or weeks). Don't wait to box and unbox your lecture until several days before an exam as it just won't work.

Students really enjoy using this technique and find that changing the box colors in their notes is a lot like playing a game with the goal of turning as many of the boxes as possible a dark green before the test. What I have seen with this technique is that the more green boxes the students have, the better they do on their exam. In fact, I have seen students begin using this technique in their classes and have their exam grades go up as much as 50%! I hope that you find this technique as helpful as they have.

Practicing Application While Studying

One of the most important goals of step 4 of the S.A.L.A.M.I. method is to make sure you can apply the information that you are learning. Being able to recall facts about specific drugs or disease states is not helpful if you can't use that knowledge to help your patients. While you do have quite a bit of control over how you can achieve learning goals 2 and 3, practicing application requires the learner to have access to practice problems. Hopefully, your instructor will provide these for you. These problem sets can come from a textbook, the instructor, or online sources.

There are several best practices that students should use when practicing application of concepts. The first is to start early and practice often. Don't make the mistake of waiting to start practicing application of concepts until you feel like you fully understand all the concepts you are studying and have fully encoded the information needed to solve the problem. Attempting to answer problem sets is a great way to enhance encoding of information and to develop a deeper understanding of concepts you are studying. Timely application practice also gives you a chance to get help from a tutor or instructors well before an assessment occurs.

The second is to attempt to simulate, exam conditions as much as possible when practicing application. There is a good chance that the practice problems your instructor assigns you will mimic the problems you might see on an examination. To simulate exam conditions, make sure you are attempting application practice without the aid of resources that are not available to you on an exam. These include notes, lecture materials, or solutions to similar types of problems as well as members of a study group. Another way to simulate exam conditions is to set a time limit for solving problems. When first starting to practice application, you are naturally going to be slower until you have had some practice. As you get closer to your assessment, you can begin to set time limits that are more realistic and in alignment with how you will need to perform on an exam. If your application practice involves mathematical calculations, make sure you are practicing with the same calculator that you will use during the exam. Many programs provide students with basic scientific calculators to use during an exam to avoid academic dishonesty. I have heard accounts from many students who could not answer problems on an exam because they were unfamiliar with how to operate the supplied calculator or because their unfamiliarity increased the time it took to calculate answers.

When practicing application by solving problem sets, many of my students fall into the trap of repeatedly solving problems without taking the time to understand the process necessary to solve the problem and without identifying the factual and theoretical information on which the problem is based. One of the ways to accomplish this is to deconstruct the problem before you attempt to solve it. Deconstruction involves the following steps:

1. Carefully read the problem and identify what the question is asking. Sometimes this can be difficult with case vignettes, especially if they are very long and detailed. If you are having difficulty with this, often the question you are being asked to answer can be found in the last two to three sentences of the case.

2. List all the major concepts related to the question. Make sure that you have some level of familiarity with each of those concepts before you attempt to an-

swer the question. After the problem has been solved, go back to your list and see if you are missing any concepts or had erroneously placed concepts in the list that are not related to the problem in question.

3. Identify information in the question that will help you to solve the problem. Being able to identify quickly pertinent information in a problem and eliminating distracting information is an important skill that can help you efficiently solve problems on exams or other assessments.

4. Determine what resources (formulas, guidelines, etc.) you will need to answer the question.

5. Determine what you will learn by answering the question. If you are having difficulty solving the problem, there is a good chance that the issue is associated with one of these steps. In addition, having this information can help a tutor or course instructor to identify quickly where you are getting stuck and to suggest a solution.

How Do I Know If I Am Ready?

I have developed a tool, a preexam checklist (Figure 8-7), to help you evaluate if you are ready for an assessment. This checklist was inspired partly by one of my childhood friends, Bill. Throughout our childhood and adult life, Bill and I have gone on many backcountry adventures. Bill is a very big picture person and is more apt to wing his way through an experience rather than meticulously plan for it. I, on the other hand, tend to obsess and worry over tiny details. We make a good pair because between the two of us we manage to plan enough to survive all our adventures and still have lots of fun in the process. When Bill was in college, he earned his private pilot's license, and, while he went on to become a successful dentist in Alaska, he still spends quite a bit of time in the air. When I fly with Bill, one of the most fascinating things to watch is his focus and meticulous attention to detail as he goes through a lengthy preflight checklist. This checklist is designed to help the pilot check the function of essential components (engine, navigation, and controls) of the aircraft before taking off. Bill was trained to fly by a retired commercial airline captain. "The Captain," as we like to call him, drilled into Bill the importance of completing the checklist and evaluating the plane and conditions before taking off. The purpose of the preexam checklist is like the preflight checklist in that it can guide you through a self-examination of your exam preparation. The checklist is designed to help you reflect on how well you prepared for your exam by reflecting on the time you devoted to exam preparation, whether you massed, blocked, or distributed practice, the types of learning materials you used, and, most importantly, the learning techniques used. In some of my classes, I have students complete this exercise during the class before the exam. I also have them make a prediction about what grade they are going to earn on the exam.

The first part of the preexam checklist asks you to set a goal for your exam grade and to make a prediction about what your exam grade will be. This prediction is important. Let's say that you predicted you would earn a 90% on an exam; but, when you got it back, you earned a 60%. In this case you have severely overestimated your grade. This is an indicator that you are overestimating what you have learned. The opposite can happen as well. As you begin to get better at tracking your learning using the results of your active recall, you should become more accurate in predicting your grade. I have found with my students that their anxiety goes down significantly when they go into an exam confident about the extent of their learning, even if they know they are not going to do well on the exam. Questions 3 and 4 in the checklist ask you about the number of hours of instruction and the number of hours that you studied. For every hour of class, you should be spending at least that much time outside of class studying. In fact, most recommendations with which I am familiar recommend anywhere from 1½ to 2 hours of study time for every hour in class. Questions 5, 6, and 7 deal with spacing. My recommendation is to space out your study and active recall in your most difficult classes every day. Make sure that enough forgetting has occurred that your active recall is challenging but not impossible. Question 8 is designed to help you reflect on the materials that you used to study. Using materials recommended by your instructor is always best. If handouts or PowerPoint® slides are provided, they are a great place to start and, in many cases, contain the most relevant and important information for learning. Do not ignore reading assignments that your instructors assign. They can provide important context for your learning and can be especially important in helping you with your preclass preparation. Question 9 deals with study groups. Study groups can be a great way to learn, provided they are productive. Unfortunately, many of my students who are in study groups often complain that they are more for social interaction than learning. If a significant amount of your study time is with a group and you are not learning as well as you would like, you may want to consider spending more time working individually. Table 8-1 can help you gauge the level of your metacognitive knowledge by identifying and rating the effectiveness of a variety of different study strategies and learning materials. The important thing to keep in mind is that you are following the guidance outlined throughout the book. If you are rereading your text over and over, if you are rereading or reviewing your notes multiple times, if you are recopying your lecture notes in an effort to absorb information, and you rate these techniques as highly effective, then please go back and read this chapter! Finally the last question asks you to rate the effectiveness of your studying. If there is a disconnection between how you rate your study and how you perform on your exam, then it is highly possible that you are suffering from a learning illusion. Check Table 8-1 and think about the strategies that you are using to learn. If they aren't evidence-based approaches, then consider changing your approach.

Figure 8-7: S.A.L.A.M.I. Method Preexam Checklist

Last Name: _____ First Name: _____

Course: _____ Exam #: _____

Introduction
The S.A.L.A.M.I. method preexam checklist is a tool designed to provide students with the opportunity to reflect on their exam preparation. The information collected in this form can be used by itself or in conjunction with an exam wrapper to make informed adjustments to course preparation and study strategies, develop exam skills, or seek assistance in reducing the impact of environmental factors on exam performance. Please answer the following questions as honestly and accurately as possible.

1. What % grade on the exam would you consider satisfactory (i.e., what is your goal)?

2. Based on your preparation, predict the % grade you will get on the exam.

3. What grade did you earn on the exam?

4. How many total hours did you spend studying for the exam?

5. Circle the statement that best describes your study pattern for this exam.

> I studied course material every day.
>
> I studied course material every other day.
>
> I studied course material 2-3 times a week.
>
> I only studied the course material right before the exam.
>
> I studied material regularly but increased the frequency, focus, and intensity right before the exam.

6. If you did not study the material every day, how many days typically passed between study sessions?

7. If you only studied material right before the exam, how many days before the exam did you start?

8. What materials did you use to study for the exam? (i.e., handouts or PowerPoint® slides provided by the instructor, self-created notes, reading assignments, other PowerPoint® slides, instructional videos/podcasts, class recordings, other). List them in order of importance.

   1.)

   2.)

   3.)

9. Did you study individually, in a group, or both? If so estimate the percentage of time spent in each.

   % time spent in individual study:

   % time spent studying with a partner or group:

10. Using the Likert scale below, rank the overall effectiveness of your exam preparation.

    Very good – 5, Good – 4, Acceptable – 3, Poor – 2, Very poor – 1

Learning Resources and Study Strategies	Est. Frequency of Use Always – 5, Most of the Time – 4, Sometimes – 3, Rarely – 2, Never – 1	Est. Effectiveness of Strategy Very Good – 5, Good – 4, Acceptable – 3, Poor – 2, Very Poor – 1
TEXTBOOK		
Reading the Text Only		
Reading & Highlighting the Text		
Reading & Taking Notes from the Text		
Rereading the Text without Taking Notes		
CLASS MATERIALS		
Reviewing/Rereading Lecture Notes or PowerPoint®		
Recopying Lecture Notes		
Attempting to Memorize Facts & Figures from Lecture Notes		
ELECTRONIC RESOURCES		
Watching Instructional Videos		
Listening to/Watching Recorded Lectures in Their Entirety		
Using Testing Apps Such as Quizlet® & Anki®		
STUDY STRATEGIES		
Self-Testing or Retrieval Practice		
Completing Assigned Problem Sets or Study Guide Questions		
Listening to/Watching Short Segments of Prerecorded Lectures		
Watching Online Tutorials		
OTHER:		

Table 8-1: A list of learning resources and study strategies that can be used to prepare for your exam. Use the Likert scales provided to indicate the frequency with which each of the resources or strategies were used and their effectiveness.

Key Concepts from Chapter 8

1. Active recall should constitute the majority of the time you spend studying.

2. There are multiple active recall strategies that can be used while studying, like focused listing, empty outline, minute paper, and the boxing technique.

3. Active recall should be done WITHOUT the aid of notes, textbooks, or other learning tools.

4. Active recall should be spaced out over time. Doing active recall directly after reviewing your notes is less effective than allowing time to pass between reviewing and self-testing.

5. Active recall should always include a self-check for the depth, breadth, and accuracy or your answer.

6. Checking the results of your active recall is a good way to gauge the extent of your learning. It can also help you plan future study sessions more effectively.

7. Any time you start to feel like you are on "autopilot" when doing active recall, it's time to mix it up. This is a sign that you are experiencing automaticity.

8. Use learning objectives from class to shape your active recall activities to match the learning expectations from your instructor.

9. Do not wait to practice application of concepts. Begin working on practice problems as soon after learning as possible.

REFERENCES

1. Nelson TO, Dunlosky J. When people's judgments of learning (JOLs) are extremely accurate at predicting subsequent recall: the "delayed-JOL effect." *Psychol Sci*. 1991;2(4):267-271.
2. Glenberg AM, Wilkinson AC, Epstein W. The illusion of knowing: failure in the self-assessment of comprehension. *Mem Cognit*. 1982;10(6):597-602. doi:10.3758/BF03202442.
3. Metcalfe J, Finn B. Evidence that judgments of learning are causally related to study choice. *Psychon Bull Rev*. 2008;15(1):174-179. doi:10.3758/PBR.15.1.174.
4. Ariel R, Dunlosky J, Bailey H. Agenda-based regulation of study-time allocation: when agendas override item-based monitoring. *J Exp Psychol Gen*. 2009;138(3):432-447. doi:10.1037/a0015928.
5. Dunlosky J. *Metacognition*. Thousand Oaks, CA: SAGE; 2008.
6. Schnee D, Ward T, Philips E, et al. Effect of live attendance and video capture viewing on student examination performance. *Am J Pharm Educ*. 2019;83(6):6897. doi:10.5688/ajpe6897.

7. Kruger J, Dunning D. Unskilled and unaware of it: how difficulties in recognizing one's own incompetence lead to inflated self-assessments. *J Pers Soc Psychol*. 1999;77(6):1121-1134. doi:10.1037/0022-3514.77.6.1121.
8. Serra MJ, DeMarree KG. Unskilled and unaware in the classroom: college students' desired grades predict their biased grade predictions. *Mem Cognit*. 2016;44(7):1127-1137. doi:10.3758/s13421-016-0624-9.
9. Hughes GI, Taylor HA, Thomas AK. Study techniques differentially influence the delayed judgment-of-learning accuracy of adolescent children and college-aged adults. *Metacognition Learn*. 2018;13(2):109-126. doi:10.1007/s11409-018-9180-y.
10. Long JD, Long EW. Enhancing student achievement through metacomprehension training. *J Dev Educ*. 1987;11(1):2-5.
11. Abott EE. On the analysis of the factor of recall in the learning process. *Psychol Rev Monogr Suppl*. 1909;11(1):159-177. doi:10.1037/h0093018.
12. Carrier M, Pashler H. The influence of retrieval on retention. *Mem Cognit*. 1992;20(6):633-642. doi:10.3758/BF03202713.
13. Bjork RA. Retrieval as a memory modifier: an interpretation of negative recency and related phenomena. In: Solso RL, ed. *Information Processing and Cognition: The Loyola Symposium*. Mahwah, NJ: Lawrence Erlbaum Associates; 1975: 123-144.
14. Roediger HL, Karpicke JD. Test-enhanced learning: taking memory tests improves long-term retention. *Psychol Sci*. 2006;17(3):249-255. doi:10.1111/j.1467-9280.2006.01693.x.
15. Bjork EL, Bjork RA. Making things hard on yourself, but in a good way: creating desirable difficulties to enhance learning. In: Gernsbacher MA, Pew RW, Hough L, Pomerantz JR, eds. *Psychology and the Real World: Essays Illustrating Fundamental Contributions to Society*. New York, NY: Worth Publishers; 2011: 56-64.
16. Cepeda NJ, Pashler H, Vul E, Wixted JT, Rohrer D. Distributed practice in verbal recall tasks: a review and quantitative synthesis. *Psychol Bull*. 2006;132(3):354-380. doi:10.1037/0033-2909.132.3.354.
17. Bahrick HP. The long-term neglect of long-term memory: reasons and remedies. In: Healy AF, ed. *Experimental Cognitive Psychology and Its Applications*. Washington, DC: American Psychological Association; 2005:89-100. doi:10.1037/10895-007.
18. Dempster FN. The spacing effect: a case study in the failure to apply the results of psychological research. *Am Psychol*. 1988;43(8):627-634. doi:10.1037/0003-066X.43.8.627.
19. Terenyi J, Anksorus H, Persky AM. Optimizing the spacing of retrieval practice to improve pharmacy students' learning of drug names. *Am J Pharm Educ*. 2019;83(6):7029. doi:10.5688/ajpe7029.
20. Karpicke JD, Bauernschmidt A. Spaced retrieval: absolute spacing enhances learning regardless of relative spacing. *J Exp Psychol Learn Mem Cogn*. 2011;37(5):1250-1257. doi:10.1037/a0023436.
21. Bjork RA, Dunlosky J, Kornell N. Self-regulated learning: beliefs, techniques, and illusions. *Annu Rev Psychol*. 2013;64(1):417-444. doi:10.1146/annurev-psych-113011-143823.
22. Miller EK, Buschman TJ. Working memory capacity: limits on the bandwidth of cognition. *Daedalus*. 2015;144(1):112-122. doi:10.1162/DAED_a_00320.
23. Karpicke JD, Blunt JR. Retrieval practice produces more learning than elaborative studying with concept mapping. *Science*. 2011;331(6018):772-775. doi:10.1126/science.1199327.
24. Blunt JR, Karpicke JD. Learning with retrieval-based concept mapping. *J Educ Psychol*. 2014;106(3):849-858. doi:10.1037/a0035934.

CHAPTER 9
S.A.L.A.M.I. Method Step 5: Postassessment Review

Case Study

P.T. is a second-year pharmacy student who has taken the third exam in the pharmacology course. Several days later, the student goes to the course's learning management system where an exam grade of 65% is posted. The student schedules a meeting with the course instructor, Dr. J.C., to review the exam. P.T. was expecting an 85%. During the meeting, the student reviews the questions that were answered incorrectly, asks several basic content-related questions, and argues for points over one answer. Fifteen minutes later, P.T. leaves Dr. J.C.'s office with the same grade and the following advice from his instructor, "You just need to study more, and you will do better on the next exam."

CASE STUDY ANALYSIS

This case describes a common interaction between a student and faculty member during exam return. Very often, exam reviews can be an unproductive investment of time and, in many cases, can be very frustrating for both parties. Why is this? I believe it is partly due to student attitudes about exams. Let's consider the following study, conducted in 2011 at Purdue University School of Pharmacy. Nearly 65% of pharmacy students who completed this survey responded that the primary purpose of an examination was to assess their level of learning. An additional 28% indicated that examinations were done primarily to assign a grade to their performance, while only 7% recognized that examinations were valuable for improving their learning.[1] These results suggest that while most pharmacy students understand the value of exams in measuring their learning, most are unaware that there are significant learning benefits from taking an exam. I hope that when you are finished with this chapter you will see what the research presents — that taking and then engaging in a structured review of the exam are valuable opportunities to learn and improve metacognition.[2-4]

Postassessment review is perhaps one of the most important steps of the S.A.L.A.M.I. method, yet it is one most likely to be skipped by students. Think about your own experience with exam return. You anxiously wait as your instructor posts grades on a course learning shell or passes exams back in class. You sit with your exam for several minutes reviewing what you got wrong, perhaps looking for questions where you might argue for a few extra points. You turn it in and never think about it again. On rare occasions, you might make an appointment with your instructor to review your exam further, especially if you did not achieve a passing grade. These strategies are extremely passive and usually provide little insight into what you truly know or how you might alter how you study to perform better in the future. Now let's consider an alternative scenario in which you engage in a structured, reflective exam review process. Using a tool called an "exam wrapper," you analyze your exam performance and generate data that can be used to make positive changes to the way that you prepare for future assessments. In this chapter, you are going to learn exactly how to do this.

I have found that many instructors and students spend very little time or energy engaging in a structured exam review that allows them to determine not only where knowledge deficiencies are but also to gain insight into how to prepare more effectively for the next assessment. This has always puzzled me as most professionals don't function in this way. For example, let's look at the teams in the National Football League (NFL), specifically what they do to evaluate their game-day performance. One of the most important weekly practice activities after a game for coaches and players is to review the game-day video and assess their performance. Based on this information, coaches can strategically adjust practices to make improvement in skills and knowledge and to prepare better for the next game. The U.S. Army uses a similar strategy referred to as the after-action review (AAR). An AAR is a structured debriefing process that allows soldiers to analyze the effectiveness of their performance in a military exercise or mission. Ultimately, this process is used to correct deficiencies, identify and sustain areas of strength, and help leaders and soldiers to focus on the performance of specific mission-essential tasks.[5] As a former combat medic, I participated in many AARs to analyze our unit's performance on mass casualty exercises and found them to be extremely useful. Fortunately, students can use a similar approach to analyze their exam preparation and performance using tool called an "exam wrapper."[6]

I have devised my own exam wrapper that is based on the four different learning goals introduced in Chapter 2 and the best practices and evidence-based approaches to studying that I have written about throughout this book. A complete copy of the exam wrapper is available with the digital edition of the book on PharmacyLibrary.com. I am going to break the exam wrapper down into its different sections and explain how you can use this tool in your own classes to improve your studying and learning.

The S.A.L.A.M.I. exam wrapper is divided into five different sections. Sections 1 through 3 are designed to determine if and how well you met the four learning goals: priming for learning, understanding and building context, memory formation and strengthening, and utilization. Section 4 is designed to help you identify any deficiencies in exam-taking skills. The last section will help you reflect on any behavioral or wellness factors that may have had an impact on your exam performance. As you read through the exam wrapper, you will see that there are a series of statements within each of the five sections. These statements are designed to help you identify specific factors that may have contributed to missing a question. To use the wrapper, begin to review your exam and identify all the questions that you missed. Then match one or more of the statements listed in each of the first four sections that best describes why you missed that question. Once you have matched statements to a missed question, record the question number next to that statement. After you have completed this for all the missed questions, add up the number of questions you have recorded in each section. Large scores in a section may indicate an issue with achieving that learning goal. This wrapper should be completed as soon as possible after your exam has been returned to you.

Section 1. Priming for Learning and Understanding and Building Context

Let's take a closer look at section 1 and what it might look like filled out. Imagine that you are reviewing a recent pharmacology exam. You missed sixteen questions and earned a 68%. As you review your exam, you realize that you missed question 3, 5, 9, and 15 because you didn't understand how ACE Inhibitors work and questions 22-26 because you missed class the day those concepts were taught. Based on this, you would fill out section 1 of the exam wrapper (Figure 9-1).

Figure 9-1: Section 1 of the Exam Wrapper

Section 1. PRIMING FOR LEARNING AND UNDERSTANDING AND BUILDING CONTEXT	Question Number
1. I had difficulty understanding concepts necessary to answer the question.	3, 5, 9, 15
2. I did not understand the relationship between 2 or more concepts (i.e., mechanism of action and clinical use, ionization and solubility, transcription and translation).	
3. I missed class the day this concept was covered and had to make up the information.	22, 23, 24, 25, 26
TOTAL SCORE:	9

SUGGESTED CORRECTIVE ACTIONS:
1. Complete previewing sheet before attending class.
2. Develop S.M.A.R.T. goals for each study session.
3. Review and analyze course and lecture learning objectives to gauge instructor's expectations for depth and breadth of learning.
4. Ensure that you are reactivating related knowledge before attending class.
5. Don't copy every word the instructor says; rather, listen and summarize main concepts.
6. Use lecture recordings to fill in gaps in your notes or to review explanation of concepts that were confusing.
7. Use the results from active recall or completed practice problems to identify gaps in your knowledge or understanding. Then get timely help from content experts (course instructors, teaching assistants, or tutors.)
8. Attend class regularly and make sure you are fully participating in active learning exercises.

The total score of 9 on section 1 (56% of questions missed) is an indicator that learning goals 1 and 2 have not been fully achieved. At the bottom of section 1 are possible corrective actions that you can take to ensure that you are able to achieve these learning goals on the next exam. Based on the reasons why you missed these nine questions, I would recommend making sure that you implement the corrective actions listed in this section. Making sure that you use the results of active recall and completion of problem sets to identify areas of difficulty and ensuring that you get timely help from content experts like faculty, teaching assistants, and tutors are important steps for avoiding these issues on the next exam.

Section 2. Memory Formation and Strengthening

Section 2 of the exam wrapper is designed to help you evaluate how well the strategies you used while studying worked to encode and consolidate information into long-term memory. Of all sections on the exam wrapper, this section seems to be the highest scoring for most of my students, especially those who are using ineffective and passive strategies like reviewing or recopying their notes. In this case, let's imagine that you are reviewing a therapeutics exam and you missed ten questions on the exam (2, 4, 7, 15, 19, 23, 27, 30, 43, and 45) and you are able to identify a specific reason for why you missed each of these questions in this section (Figure 9-2).

Figure 9-2: Section 2 of the Exam Wrapper.

Section 2. **MEMORY FORMATION AND STRENGTHENING**	Question Number
1. I studied but could not recall **any** of the facts and concepts needed to answer the question.	2, 4, 7, 43, 45
2. I recalled **some** of the facts and concepts to answer the question but not all of them.	15, 19, 23, 27
3. I recalled the facts and concepts to answer the question but not in **enough detail.**	30
4. I struggled to remember facts and information quickly.	
5. I did not study the material necessary to answer the question.	43, 45
TOTAL SCORE:	**12**

SUGGESTED CORRECTIVE ACTIONS:
1. Use active recall strategies when preparing for an exam. Active recall should constitute most of your study sessions.
2. Use the results of your active recall sessions to guide future study. If using the boxing technique, pay particular attention to yellow and red boxes.
3. Avoid cramming or blocking your study. Study and practice retrieval at regularly spaced, daily intervals.
4. Interleave related subjects within your study sessions.
5. Identify and avoid distractors while studying to maintain focus and productivity.
6. Develop S.M.A.R.T. goals for each study session.
7. Review and analyze course and lecture learning objectives to gauge instructor's expectations for depth and breadth of learning.

You will notice in this case that your total score in this section is 12, even though you only missed ten questions. This score can be explained because there were multiple reasons for two of the questions missed, 43 and 45. High scores in section 2 of the exam wrapper are very common and are a strong indicator that you are not consistently and correctly using the evidence-based strategies that we have already discussed like active recall, spacing, and interleaving. Correcting this problem involves identifying what passive strategies you are using and replacing them with the evidence-based ones.

Section 3. Utilization

Section 3 of the exam wrapper is designed to help you reflect on your ability to apply, analyze, synthesize, and evaluate information you have learned. It is filled out in the same way as the first two sections (Figure 9-3).

Figure 9-3: Section 3 of the Exam Wrapper

Section 3. UTILIZATION	Question Number
1. I did not understand how to solve the problem.	
2. I had difficulty analyzing information in the question.	
3. I could not interpret a diagram, graph, table, or figure in the question.	
4. I was unable to apply facts and information to solve the problem.	
5. I was unable to make a connection between two different concepts to answer the question correctly.	
6. I made a mathematical error in my calculation.	
7. I did not have time before the exam to complete practice questions or problem sets.	
8. I lacked a general problem-solving strategy or approach that would have helped me to answer this question.	
TOTAL SCORE:	

SUGGESTED CORRECTIVE ACTIONS:
1. Ensure that you start working on assigned problems sets or questions as early as possible.
2. Get timely help from course faculty or tutors to ensure you know how to apply information.
3. Do not use notes or example problems when working on practice questions.
4. If possible, use the same calculator for practice and the exam.
5. When answering practice questions or problems, solutions should be cross-checked with reliable sources.

I have found that students scoring high in this section may have one or more of the following issues. They may not understand or have fully encoded information needed to solve the exam problems. They may have waited until right before the exam to begin completing practice problems because they found themselves cramming or were hesitant to begin trying practice problems until they had developed a perfect understanding of the material. Remember that spacing your study out over time is one of the most effective evidence-based learning strategies and it is never too early to start practicing application! In fact, many of the best instructors employ active learning and problem-solving exercises in class when teaching new concepts to get their students started on this as early as possible. Another common mistake that I see with my students is that they habitually use their notes, similar example problems, or work with other students when attempting to solve problems. Your mindset when solving any type of problem is that you should simulate exam conditions as closely as possible. Will you have your notes or be able to discuss a problem's solution with other students as you are taking an exam? Probably not. If that is the case, then don't practice that way. Think of completing practice problems like a scrimmage or dress rehearsal. If you forget your lines during a dress rehearsal, it's okay to go back and look at the script; but, when it's time for opening night, you won't have that luxury.

Another challenge students face is that their instructors may not assign practice problems or, if they do, only a small number. If this is the case, you may have to identify alternative sources for practicing the application of concepts. Before you do this, ask your instructors if they have any additional practice problems or if they can recommend a source of additional practice problems that you can use in preparing for the exam. Often the textbook that you are using or other related textbooks or workbooks that are not being used in the course are great sources for practice problems. Other good sources are board exam–review books or old copies of exams that your instructor has released for practice purposes. With a little patience and luck, you might even be able to locate practice problems online.

Many students with whom I work are afraid to ask their course instructors for help because they don't want to appear unintelligent. While these feelings can be hard to manage, you must work to overcome them. If you isolate yourself from your instructor, you are removing a critical resource for your learning. In a very short time you are going to be directly caring for patients, and any knowledge deficits you have accumulated can become a real danger to them. Keep in mind that course instructors are always the best resource to call on if you are having difficulty applying information. Many instructors can seem intimidating but are usually very willing to help if asked, especially if you schedule an appointment ahead of time or stop by during office hours prepared with specific questions and problems that you would like to review. Additionally, a short follow-up e-mail thanking them for their time can help to smooth the road for the next time you need help! If your course instructor is not an option, then I would recommend seeking out help from teaching assistants, tutors, or other students that are doing well in the course.

Section 4. Exam Skills

Section 4 of the exam wrapper deals with exam skills. Successfully learning how to navigate exams is a significant challenge for most students; yet, there is a real lack of empirical research identifying the skills, behaviors, and approaches of effective test takers. Most of it is based purely on anecdotal experience or common sense than anything else. Yet, I do strongly believe that there are certain traps into which students can fall that can have an impact on exam performance. Let's look through the nine statements about exam skills in this section of the wrapper (Figure 9-4). I have loosely grouped these statements into 3 general categories: reading errors, question analysis, and time management.

Figure 9-4: Section 4 of the Exam Wrapper

Section 4. EXAM SKILLS	Question Number
READING ERRORS	
1. I did not carefully read all answer options and picked the first one that looked correct.	
2. I read the question quickly and missed important details, meaning, or key words like "never," "always," "except," etc.	
QUESTION ANALYSIS	
3. I changed my answer and my first choice was correct.	
4. I did not understand the question.	
5. I overthought and missed what the question was asking.	
6. I did not think logically about the question.	
TIME MANAGEMENT	
7. I ran out of time and guessed at the end.	
8. I only read part of the question before choosing my answer.	
9. I did not use the process of elimination to help me to answer the question.	
TOTAL SCORE:	

SUGGESTED CORRECTIVE ACTIONS:
1. Take the first five minutes of an exam to familiarize yourself with question types. Be strategic about what questions you answer first and how much time you spend on each question.
2. Highlight key words and phrases in the question stem.
3. Familiarize yourself with the answer selections before reading the stem and attempting to answer the question.
4. Use the process of elimination to help improve your chances of getting the problem correct.
5. *Only* change your answer on a previous question if you suddenly remember or discover information in another question that might help answer a previous one.

Reading Errors

While working with students on exam analysis, I have found several common reading mistakes. Many of my students simply read questions too quickly and miss key words or important information necessary to identify the correct answer. They report doing this because of concerns about running out of time or simply forgetting information before they can answer the question. My recommendation for beating this issue is to practice as many multiple-choice questions as you can. Most time limits for multiple choice exams are based on the rule that a student should take 60 to 90 seconds to answer each question. When practicing, set a time limit for each question based on this rule and focus on reading questions carefully, identifying key words or phrases like "always," "choose the best answer," "never," and "except."

Another common reading issue I see is when my students choose the first answer that looks correct without reading all the selections. The solution to this problem is to slow down and carefully read and consider each answer choice. This is also a great time to begin to use the process of elimination to reduce the number of answers from which to choose. In extreme cases, in which I have had a student who could not break this behavior, I had that student practice reading all the answer choices first, before even reading the question.

Question Analysis

Some multiple-choice questions, especially case vignettes, may include extraneous information that is not necessary to answer the questions. Getting fixated on this information is easy, and the student can either become overwhelmed or go down a path that leads to the wrong answer. Let's look at the following sample question as an example:

M.D. is a 55-year-old, white male with a medical history of GERD, hypertension, and dyslipidemia. M.D. is taking the following medications:
Lovastatin, 20mg
Omeprazole, 20 mg
Lisinopril, 10 mg
He reports that he is compliant with all his medicines and that his GERD symptoms have subsided significantly. At the time of his appointment, M.D.'s lipid panel reveals the following:
Total cholesterol: 280 mg/dl
LDL: 168 mg/dl
HDL: 35 mg/dl
Triglycerides: 220 mg/dl

His blood pressure is 160/98. What changes should be made to M.D.'s antihypertensive drug regimen?
a) Increase his dose of lisinopril.
b) Switch M.D. to verapamil.
c) Add hydrochlorothiazide to the current regimen.
d) Continue with current therapy and reevaluate at the next visit.

There is a lot of information in this question, but only some of it is relevant and important. With a rather long, case-vignette-based question like this, I always recommend that students find and read the question stem, which is usually the last sentence in the question before anything else. This strategy will allow you to clearly identify what the question is up front. In this case the question simply is what changes should be made to M.D.'s antihypertensive drug regimen? Armed with this information, you can now begin eliminating extraneous information and focus on only the information needed to answer the question. For this question, important information would include his current blood pressure and the medication and current dose that he is taking for his hypertension. M.D. is on a relatively low dose of lisinopril, and his blood pressure is uncontrolled. Lisinopril is an appropriate medication and with the low dose there is room to titrate up. Be careful not to fixate on the dyslipidemia issue. While it is true that his lipids could be better managed, that is not what the question is asking. Unfortunately, students can get fixated on this becoming frustrated if they don't see an answer to a question that is not even being asked!

I have also seen students unconsciously "edit" the question while reading, ultimately forcing it to ask something else than what it does. This often happens when test takers get fixated on distracting and irrelevant information in the question. As an example, let's pretend that in the above example one of the answers focused on using a different statin to manage his dysipidemia. If a student didn't carefully identify what the question is asking and became fixated on the patient's lipid panel and statin, the student may focus an answer on this issue, rather than addressing the patient's blood pressure control.

Time Management

Running out of time on an exam is a common challenge for students. There are many reasons that this can happen. Let's consider some examples that I see frequently.

First, it is always a good idea to take a few minutes at the beginning of any exam to see what you are up against and to develop a basic plan. The plan may vary from exam to exam based on the content, length, and type of questions. For example, let's say you are taking a two-hour pharmacotherapeutics exam. When you begin the exam, you notice that it contains 25 multiple-choice questions, worth 50 points total, and two patient case scenarios, each worth 25 points. You quickly do some mental math to determine how much time it should take to complete the multiple-choice section of the test. Taking the 60 to 90 second/question rule, I would leave about 40 minutes to complete these questions. You also want a buffer of time at the end of the exam to clean up any unanswered questions and to ensure that you have completed everything. Conservatively, I would recommend about 15 minutes for that. That means you have about an hour to complete both cases and I would recommend starting those first. They are going to take the most amount of time to answer and cannot be rushed through at the end of the exam, especially if you are running out of time. Multiple-choice questions can typically be answered more quickly, and it is much better to leave a few unanswered than an entire essay question incomplete.

Students that have used the passive, ineffective learning strategies that I have described throughout this book may have difficulty quickly and accurately remembering information needed to answer a question. This may be caused by what is referred to as storage and retrieval strength. Generally defined, retrieval strength is a measure of how quickly we can recall information when needed, and storage strength is an indicator of how well learned or encoded information is in long-term memory.[7] To combat these problems, I have several recommendations. The first is to make sure that your studying includes lots of spaced, active recall. This is the best way to increase the probability that you can quickly and accurately remember information that you need to answer questions. The second is to work on a lot of practice problems. When doing practice problems, make sure you attempt to complete them under timed conditions and without the aid of your notes. Working under these conditions will increase the probability that you can complete problems successfully on the exam. Thirdly, if you find yourself stuck on a multiple-choice question for more than about 3 minutes, mark it and move on.

Section 5. Behavioral and Wellness Factors

This last section of the exam wrapper (Figure 9-5) is a little different from the first four. It contains seven different statements about distraction, test anxiety, and wellness. Unlike the previous four sections, you are not matching a missed question to one of these statements, rather you respond to each statement with a yes or no answer. Take a few minutes to read through the statements and the possible corrective actions below.

Figure 9-5: Section 5 of the Exam Wrapper

Section 5. BEHAVIORAL AND WELLNESS FACTORS Answer YES or NO	YES or NO
1. I was distracted by noise or other students during the exam.	
2. I had a difficult time focusing and concentrating during the exam.	
3. I blanked on information necessary to answer questions.	
4. I felt anxious during this exam and felt that had an impact on my grade.	
5. I froze during the exam.	
6. I did not sleep well or got enough sleep the night before the exam.	
7. I did not appropriately eat and hydrate before the exam.	

SUGGESTED CORRECTIVE ACTIONS
1. If approved by proctors, utilize ear plugs to help eliminate distractions from noise.
2. Get enough sleep before the exam.
3. Eat and hydrate properly before the exam begins.
4. Seek out assistance from professional sources (academic affairs office, disability support, or campus counseling services) if you suspect that you have a learning disability or severe exam anxiety.
5. Use time limits when practicing problems to simulate exam conditions and make sure that spaced, active recall is a major strategy that you use during study.

DISTRACTION

Having proctored hundreds of exams over the last twenty years, I can attest that even under the best test conditions, there still is going to be some level of background noise that may be distracting to students. Any time you pack many students into a room there is going to be noise from students dropping things, shuffling papers, getting up after completing the exam, coughing, sneezing, and asking exam proctors questions. For some students, these noises can break their concentration or make them anxious. One possible solution for this problem is to wear foam ear plugs during the exam. If you decide to try this solution, please check with your exam proctors to ensure that this is allowed. If the earplugs don't work or the issue is so serious that it is having a significant impact on your grade, I encourage you to schedule an appointment with your Disability Support Services Office. You may be eligible for examination accommodations. Over the years I have taught or coached students for whom this was a serious problem, and exam accommodations that include a reduced distraction environment made all the difference.

TEST ANXIETY

In early 2021, Pate and colleagues published an important multiinstitutional study looking at test anxiety in pharmacy students. What they discovered was very compelling. A total of 124 pharmacy students from three different schools of pharmacy completed a validated, self-reporting tool designed to measure test anxiety. Of the 119 student results analyzed, 18.5 % of students reported having high test anxiety and 34.5 % reported having moderate test anxiety. Even more surprising was the effect that this anxiety had on academic success. Students that reported having a high degree of test anxiety generally had a much lower total scaled score on the NAPLEX. They also had lower cumulative grade point averages (GPAs) and Pharmacy Curriculum Outcomes Assessment (PCOA) scores and were more likely to need remediation in their courses.[8] These numbers also correlate well to other studies in different student populations demonstrating similar rates of test anxiety and resulting academic difficulties.[9-12]

Students who suffer from test anxiety may experience a wide range of physical, emotional, and cognitive symptoms including elevated heart rate, dizzyness, nausea, or even panic. Emotionally, students may also feel worried and constantly engage in comparing their academic performance to their peers. They may be fixated on failing exams or courses and what will happen as a result. They may be worried about letting down their parents and teachers and consistently lack confidence in their exam preparation.[13,14]

Significant test anxiety can also impair your ability to prepare effectively for an exam, interfering with your ability to encode and retrieve information during study needed to answer exam questions.[15,16]

Keep in mind that while most students experience preexam jitters or nervousness, true test anxiety can be crippling and has a significant impact on learning and exam performance. If you are experiencing anxiety symptoms that you believe are having an impact on your ability to learn and to perform well on exams, I encourage you to seek out help from a mental health care provider. There are many approaches and techniques that can be used to help reduce or eliminate this anxiety. A good place to start is your campus counseling center. The health care professionals staffing these centers more than likely have a great deal of experience helping students to manage this condition. In addition, there is evidence that retrieval practice has been shown to reduce anxiety in students taking exams.[17] Many of the students that use the boxing technique I discussed in Chapter 8 report feeling less anxious because they have actual data in the form of colored boxes that can show them how much they know prior to the exam. If they have a lot of green boxes, they report being more confident and less anxious about how they are going to perform.

I hope that you can see that using a tool like the S.A.L.A.M.I. method exam wrapper can help you to analyze your exam preparation and performance in a structured way. The data that you collect from the exam wrapper is no good unless you reflect on it and use it to make changes to the way that you prepare for and take your next exam. Comparing the results of exam wrappers from multiple exams and across courses can tell you whether challenges you face are course specific or are more generalized across the curriculum. Always remember that the number one, best strategy for taking an exam is to make sure that you are properly prepared. If you have used the evidence-based approaches discussed throughout this book and ensured that you know how to use the information you have learned in the way that your instructor expects, you should be able to avoid many of the problems discussed in this book.

Key Concepts from Chapter 9

1. **Examinations are not just important opportunities to determine what you know. They are important learning opportunities.**

2. **Structured exam review using an exam wrapper can provide insight into the effectiveness of your preparation and important clues for how you might need to change your approach to studying.**

3. **Test anxiety can have a significant negative impact on your ability to perform well on assessments. If you suspect that this may be an issue, mental health support services and test accommodations can be extremely helpful.**

4. **Failure is a natural and necessary part of learning. A productive response to a bad test grade is essential to avoid a repeat performance on a subsequent exam.**

5. **Don't try to fix the problem on your own! Most schools have a number of academic support resources that can help you to improve your learning. These include course instructors, academic advisors, tutors, student affairs personnel, tutors, and campus learning centers.**

REFERENCES

1. Hagemeier NE, Mason HL. Student pharmacists' perceptions of testing and study strategies. *Am J Pharm Educ*. 2011;75(2):35. doi:10.5688/ajpe75235.
2. Medina MS, Castleberry AN, Persky AM. Strategies for improving learner metacognition in health professional education. *Am J Pharm Educ*. 2017;81(4):78. doi:10.5688/ajpe81478.
3. Roediger III HL, Putnam AL, Smith MA. Ten benefits of testing and their applications to educational practice. In: Mestre JP, Ross BH, eds. *The Psychology of Learning and Motivation: Cognition in Education, Vol. 55*. New York, NY: Elsevier Academic Press; 2011:1-36. doi:10.1016/B978-0-12-387691-1.00001-6.
4. Marsh EJ, Roediger HL, Bjork RA, Bjork EL. The memorial consequences of multiple-choice testing. *Psychon Bull Rev*. 2007;14(2):194-199. doi:10.3758/BF03194051.
5. Zajtchuk R, Bellamy RF, eds. *War Psychiatry*. Washington, DC: Office of The Surgeon General at TMM Publications; 1995.
6. Lovett MC. Make exams worth more than the grade: using exam wrappers to promote metacognition. In: Kaplan M, Silver N, LaVaque-Manty D, Meizlish D, eds. *Using Reflection and Metacognition to Improve Student Learning: Across the Disciplines, Across the Academy*. Sterling, VA: Stylus Publishing, LLC; 2013: 18-52.
7. Bjork RA, Bjork EL. A new theory of disuse and an old theory of stimulus fluctuation. In: F. Healy FA, Kosslyn SM, Shiffrin RM, eds. *Essays in Honor of William K. Estes, Vol. 1. From Learning Theory to Connectionist Theory, Vol. 2*. From Learning Processes to Cognitive Processes. Mahwah, NJ: Lawrence Erlbaum Associates, Inc.; 1992:35-67.
8. Pate AN, Neely S, Malcom DR, Daugherty KK, Zagar M, Medina MS. Multisite study assessing the effect of cognitive test anxiety on academic and standardized test performance. *Am J Pharm Educ*. 2021;85(1):8041. doi:10.5688/ajpe8041.
9. Putwain D, Daly AL. Test anxiety prevalence and gender differences in a sample of English secondary school students. *Educ Stud*. 2014;40(5):554-570. doi:10.1080/03055698.2014.953914.
10. Thomas CL, Cassady JC, Finch WH. Identifying severity standards on the cognitive test anxiety scale: cut score determination using latent class and cluster analysis. *J Psychoeduc Assess*. 2018;36(5):492-508. doi:10.1177/0734282916686004.
11. von der Embse N, Jester D, Roy D, Post J. Test anxiety effects, predictors, and correlates: a 30-year meta-analytic review. *J Affect Disord*. 2018;227(2):483-493. doi:10.1016/j.jad.2017.11.048.
12. Cassady JC, Johnson RE. Cognitive test anxiety and academic performance. *Contemp Educ Psychol*. 2002;27(2):270-295. doi:10.1006/ceps.2001.1094.
13. Deffenbacher JL, Hazaleus SL. Cognitive, emotional, and physiological components of test anxiety. *Cogn Ther Res*. 1985;9(2):169-180. doi:10.1007/BF01204848.
14. Hembree R, College A. Correlates, causes, effects, and treatment of test anxiety. *Rev Educ Res*. 1988;58(1):47-77.
15. Rohrer D, Taylor K. The effects of overlearning and distributed practise on the retention of mathematics knowledge. *Appl Cogn Psychol*. 2006;20(9):1209-1224. doi:10.1002/acp.1266.
16. Dougherty KM, Johnston JM. Overlearning, fluency, and automaticity. *Behav Anal*. 1996; 19(2):289-292. doi:10.1007/BF03393171.
17. Agarwal PK, D'Antonio L, Roediger HL, McDermott KB, McDaniel MA. Classroom-based programs of retrieval practice reduce middle school and high school students' test anxiety. *J Appl Res Mem Cogn*. 2014;3(3):131-139. doi:10.1016/j.jarmac.2014.07.002.

CHAPTER 10
Final Thoughts

I wrap up this book with a few thoughts on a topic we have not yet discussed: how to effectively respond to an academic crisis. Perhaps you just underperformed on a major assessment or maybe you are doing poorly in one or more courses. If so, what steps can you take to maximize the chances that you can turn things around? The first thing to remember is that student learning can be influenced by many different factors. In 1993, Hartman and Sternberg published a paper describing a comprehensive model of learning including the many different factors that influence student academic performance called the B A C E I S model (Behavior, Affect, Cognition, Environment, Interacting, Systems).[1] This model has been highly influential in my thinking about student success, and I believe that components of this model can be useful to students.

Identifying the issues that have an impact on your learning is critical as the strategies you used to improve your learning and performance should be focused on eliminating or reducing the impact of negative factors. For example, if you believe that your learning difficulties are based on an inability to self-regulate your learning, a lack of metacognition, poor study or productivity skills, or problems with motivation, then this book could be a useful tool.

If, however, you suspect that external factors are contributing to your academic difficulties such as physical or mental health issues, a learning disability, family or relationship issues, or financial challenges, you will need to seek support from other sources.[2]

Crisis Management

As a student, I had my share of bad exam performances. Prior to my introduction to effective study strategies, my response to a bad exam grade could be categorized in three ways:

Response 1. Panic and promise myself that I would simply study harder for the next exam.

Response 2. Panic and convince myself that this exam grade was just a fluke and the next one would be better.

Response 3. Give up, believing that the grade I received was the best of which I was capable.

Perhaps some of you can relate to these responses. Looking back, I can confidently tell you that none of them were productive or helped to improve my learning. Hopefully, if you made it this far in the book, you realize this as well.

So how should you respond to a bad test performance? Responding appropriately and quickly to a bad exam grade is essential for good academic performance. Here are some tips to ensure that your response is both timely and productive.

TIP 1. ALLOW YOURSELF TIME TO PROCESS YOUR EMOTIONS.

Most students receiving an unexpected bad exam grade experience several negative emotions. Theses emotions can range from confusion and anger to self-doubt and anxiety. Allowing yourself to feel these emotions and process them is important. All these emotions are entirely normal responses to failure. Acknowledging them is an important step in moving forward in a productive way. Processing negative emotions can sometimes take time. While giving yourself this time is important, you should not allow yourself to be paralyzed by them. Remember, with appropriate academic support, strong metacognitive awareness, and an effective study strategy, you can overcome most challenges. Processing any negative emotions before you seek help from your instructors is also important. The attitude and focus that you bring to a meeting with your instructor can be the difference between one that is productive and one that is destructive.

TIP 2. SEEK OUT ASSISTANCE ASAP (AS SOON AS POSSIBLE).

Denial about poor course performance is a common student pitfall. I have worked with many students who wait until 75% of the semester is completed before coming to me for help. When I asked why they didn't come to see me sooner, the most common response I get is "I thought I could fix the problem on my own." Don't make this mistake. Most courses are structured in a way that requires students to master basic material before they move on to more complex topics. These courses can move fast, and you can quickly find yourself significantly behind. In addition, it takes time and effort to learn about, apply, and benefit from the strategies and approaches in this book. Most students I coach require several meetings with me before their academic performance begins to improve. The sooner you get help, the sooner you can start implementing strategies and behaviors that allow you to monitor and regulate your learning in a positive way. Academic assistance can be found with your course instructors, tutors, your student affairs staff, learning centers, and campus counseling. If you have these resources, use them!

TIP 3. PREPARE FOR YOUR MEETING WITH YOUR INSTRUCTOR.

Whether meeting with your instructor to ask questions about course content or to review an exam, make sure you are prepared for your meeting. Having the appropriate course materials with you and a list of specific questions can go a long way in making your meeting more productive. If you are meeting with your instructor to review an exam, ask if using the S.A.L.A.M.I. method exam wrapper to help you evaluate your performance would be possible. If your instructor is unfamiliar or unsure about exam wrappers, send your instructor a copy to look at before your meeting. Be prepared to explain the purpose of the exam wrapper, what you hope to learn from it, and how you plan to use that information to improve your learning of the material and subsequent exam performance. In your meeting, focus on wanting to understand more clearly your instructor's expectations for learning. Make it clear that, while you are concerned about your performance in the course, you understand that your score is an indicator you are not learning effectively or focusing on the right material. Keep in mind that no instructor likes to hear the question, "What do we need to know for the exam?" or to spend time arguing with students looking for a few extra points.

TIP 4. USE AVAILABLE RESOURCES IN- AND OUTSIDE OF YOUR INSTITUTION.

In some cases, "self-diagnosis and treatment" of poor academic performance is not going to be enough to fix the academic difficulties you are having, and you may need to get some external help. If you are unsure of where to go, I would suggest starting with your school or college of pharmacy's Office of Student Affairs. These offices are staffed with personnel who will be able to help you directly or point you to relevant institutional resources such as student learning centers. Staff in these learning centers may include academic coaches and tutors who can help guide you through the process of becoming a more effective learner. Hopefully, they will be aware of evidence-based learning strategies, can teach you how to use them, and understand how to evaluate and improve your metacognitive awareness.

If your university or college lacks the aforementioned resources or you have found them to be ineffective, I have some suggestions for external resources that you may find helpful. I strongly encourage you to check out Dr. Barbara Oakley and Dr. Terry Sejnowski's Massive Online Open Course "Learning How to Learn" available at **https://www.coursera.org/learn/learning-how-to-learn**. I have taken their course and found it to be heavily based on the science of learning, well-organized, well-presented, and informative. It does take some time to get through, but the effort is well worth it. If you are the type of student that does not want to go it alone, I would recommend checking out the folks at STATMed Learning at **https://statmedlearning.com**. STATMed Learning founder, Ryan Orwig, is a learning specialist with over twenty years of experience working with struggling health professions students of all types to help them to learn more effectively and pass board certification exams. I have worked with him and his team for over ten years and can attest to the quality of their evidence-based approach to teaching students how to study and take exams.

One of the most important lessons about academic success that I have learned and the final one that I would like to share with you is that persistence is the key to success. Each fall our school holds a P-1 Success Week. Scheduled directly after our first-year student's initial set of exams, this week is structured to help students become more effective independent learners through productivity, study strategies, and metacognitive development. On the first day, I show my students a TEDxBYU talk given by Eduardo Zanatta entitled, "Failure Is a Part of Success." In this talk, Mr. Zanatta discusses three principles that allow us to use failure to our advantage. One of those principles I find particularly useful is based on some excellent advice that he learned from a former professor, "Get in line and stay in line." I love this statement, and it is one that my students and I repeat over and over again. Once you get into pharmacy school, perseverance is the key. Work smart, use your resources, and immerse yourself in the experience. If you run into challenges, my advice is don't quit! With guidance and encouragement, students can achieve a lot more than they realize, and there is nothing more rewarding for me than to watch a student achieve full potential through hard work and determination.

I hope the systematic, evidence-based approach to learning I have presented to you in this book is helpful, whether you choose to use the whole method or just the parts that make sense to you. I also hope you have learned that there is a science behind learning which you can use to become a more effective, independent learner. Remember that authentic learning is never easy, but it is always rewarding, and those rewards will pay off for the rest of your life.

REFERENCES

1. Hartman H, Sternberg RJ. A broad BACEIS for improving thinking. *Instr Sci*. 1993;21:401-425. https://doi.org/10.1007/BF00121204.
2. Wittstrom KM, Godwin DA, Bleske BE. Intervention and remediation: a descriptive study of practices in pharmacy education. *Curr Pharm Teach Learn*. 2021;13(3):206-212. doi:10.1016/j.cptl.2020.10.012.